One Foot in Heaven

Journey of a Hospice Nurse

Heidi Telpner, R.N.

Contents

Author Note

The stories are true. Names, locations and certain details have been changed to protect patient confidentiality.

What is a Hospice?

Hospice, in the earliest days, was a concept rooted in the centuries-old idea of offering a place of shelter and rest, or "hospitality" to weary and sick travelers on a long journey. Dame Cicely Saunders at St. Christopher's Hospice in London first applied the term "hospice" to specialized care for dying patients in 1967. Today, hospice care provides humane and compassionate care for people in the last phases of incurable disease so that they may live as fully and comfortably as possible.

Hospice is a philosophy of care. The hospice philosophy recognizes death as the final stage of life and seeks to enable patients to continue an alert, pain-free life and to manage other symptoms so that their last days may be spent with dignity and quality, surrounded by their loved ones. Hospice affirms life and does not hasten or postpone death. Hospice care treats the person rather than the disease; it highlights quality rather than length of life. It provides family-centered care involving the patient and family in making decisions. Care is provided for the patient and family 24 hours a day, 7 days a week. Hospice care can be given in the patient's home, a hospital, nursing home, or private hospice facility. Most hospice care in the United States is given in the home, with a family member or members serving as the main hands-on caregiver.

The American Cancer Society

Introduction

There's always a beginning, whether we realize it or not. My beginning happened long before I ever interviewed for a position with hospice or ever considered the possibility of entering nursing school. Shortly after my sixteenth birthday I was in a serious horseback riding accident. I nearly died.

Who knows? It's entirely possible I was drawn to hospice because of my own near death experience. However, that's not why I'm a nurse. I became a nurse because the original plan for my life didn't pan out.

I majored in English at the University of Iowa. The plan was to publish my first novel by the age of twenty-five, be a complete degenerate by the time I turned thirty and dead long before I was over the hill at forty. Unfortunately, although I managed to get some poetry and articles published, my first novel was rejected. I found I had little interest in teaching, but with an English degree I wasn't qualified for much else. My college roommate had been in nursing school. I frequently helped her prep for her tests and along the way discovered that her classes interested me. Since I had nothing better to do at the time, I completely shocked everyone who knew me by applying to nursing school. The biggest shock of all was that I liked it.

My first real area of interest, my calling if you will, was obstetrical nursing. I still love it. Every aspect of pregnancy and the birth process amazes me. Each birth I attended during my training reduced me to tears. I even apprenticed briefly with a lay midwife in Utah. I intended to apply to the Frontier School of Midwifery in Kentucky after graduation and it was my dream to spend the rest of my life birthin' babies. However, a quickie marriage, a baby of my own delivered by a midwife, a divorce that left me without any financial support whatsoever and looming government student loan payments forced me to make an abrupt change in plans. After graduation I got the highest paying job I could find. I took a position as a staff nurse in the Intensive Care Unit of a regional Trauma Center.

I'm a quick study. Within eight months, I'd been promoted to Night Charge Nurse for the ten-bed Coronary Care Unit, managing both cardiac patients and overseeing another ten-bed Intensive Care Unit. I also monitored the Telemetry Unit and covered Codes throughout the hospital. In addition, I scheduled staffing for our after-hours Recovery Room and became the hospital's official IV-starter.

My first months of trauma care were an adrenaline junkie's dream. Between working nights and single-parenting an active toddler, sleep didn't really factor into my life. At the time I didn't mind because I considered myself part of a special breed of health care providers. We were doctors and nurses who could look serious injury and death in the face every day yet leave the hospital in a good mood. In fact, the more trauma patients the staff handled successfully, the better our collective mood at the end of a shift. By necessity, immunity from emotional distress came with the job description.

In my defense, I was young and like almost everyone else I worked with, caught up in the crazy business of keeping people alive. Frankly, I didn't have time to get attached to my patients. I'm not entirely certain I even saw them as people. They were more like a set of complicated systems. At the start of my shift I'd break every patient down into a series of tasks and assign staff accordingly. It was the simplest and most effective way to keep each set of systems running. That was my job, to keep systems, or rather, patients alive long enough to get them out of my unit so I could receive the next admission. If patients didn't transfer to the step-down unit, it was because he or she Coded and died.

As Charge Nurse I deliberately assigned myself the most complicated patients on the Unit because I enjoyed the challenge. I took exceptional care of everyone. It's funny that to this day I still remember the most difficult procedures I performed, both on my own and those I assisted with, but I can't recall a single patient's name.

The suffering, the deaths and even the success stories were never personal. I took them all in stride. We very often cared for people who had suffered horrific injury, illness and loss. "Personal" would have made my job impossible. "Personal" would have traumatized me. I figured out pretty quickly how to compartmentalize in order to survive. For better or for worse it seemed to come naturally to me. I made every effort to leave my work behind the closed doors of the hospital. After all, I had a young son depending on me to be a normal mom during my off hours.

In four years of deaths only a single one really got under my skin. It was an extraordinary experience, something I carry with me every day. I assigned myself a gentleman who had been diagnosed with pancreatic cancer. He landed in Coronary Care because we had an empty bed and Med/Surg, the Medical-Surgical Unit, was full. Pancreatic cancer is nearly always a death sentence. Death usually comes quickly, although I've since managed a number of hospice patients who survived as long as five years after experimental treatment before the disease caught up with them.

Early in the morning, after I had worked a grueling double shift, this very polite gentleman Coded. His situation was unusual because according to the monitor and my stethoscope he had no heartbeat, yet he lay there wide awake, talking to me. I hit the Code button and the team came running.

At that moment, the patient's own physician walked into the Unit on rounds. He waved off the Emergency

Room doctor and elected to run the Code himself. All through CPR and repeated shocks, the patient continued to speak and I repeatedly apologized for hurting him. While he seemed unaffected by our actions, I was in agony. I had never Coded anyone who was conscious. Ultimately, beneath my chest compressions, this man's sternum broke clean away from his ribs and remained depressed. I burst into tears. I could not continue the Code and informed the doctor.

He shrugged and said, "Call it then," and strolled nonchalantly from the room. Everyone else packed it in and left.

The poor man was still awake. The monitor reading showed his heart at seven ventricular beats a minute. For those of you unfamiliar with the way the heart works, that's pretty much dead. I got down on my knees beside the bed, leaned my head close to his, and whispered, "I am so, so sorry."

He laid a weak hand on my shoulder and said, very clearly, "Don't worry. I'm no longer in my body. I didn't feel any of it. I've been floating up here near the ceiling watching you all work."

I sat back on my heels for a moment, pretty choked up. While his words didn't surprise me because I'd once been in his position, I was overcome with awe and could barely speak.

My voice shaking, but ever the pragmatist, I finally croaked out, "Well, let's get all this stuff off of you and give you a bath. The least I can do is send you to heaven clean."

He replied, "Thank you." Those were the man's final words to me.

Though my shift had ended an hour before, I waved the day nurse away and stayed with him myself. I bathed him gently, covered him with a clean gown and then I pulled up a chair and held his hand until he died. He took his time. After a while he sighed and left his body.

You can always tell when someone dies because up until the very moment of death, up until the millisecond a person leaves his body, he or she is still present. I guess I would describe the phenomenon by saying that you can literally see someone inhabit their body because you can watch them leave it behind. The instant the person dies, but not a moment before, every cell gives up the ghost, or the soul, or the spirit, or whatever you choose to call it and the body grows waxy and lightless.

To me it seems obvious that the body is a shell, a wonderful machine built to house the soul. There's a *Star Trek* episode entitled "Spock's Brain," in which aliens remove Mr. Spock's brain and use it to power their environmental systems. Thanks to Dr. McCoy, Spock's body lives on as a soulless automaton until his brain is reattached. That's the body. However, another *Star Trek* episode may be even more descriptive of death. Its title is, "That Which Survives." In this episode, Ensign Wyatt, one of the Enterprise's typical expendable crewmen, dies in the transporter room because the holographic projection of a woman touches him. After examining the body, Dr. McCoy says, "It's as if every cell in his body's been disrupted, Jim." That's death. The soul inhabits every single cell and death disrupts every one of them.

In my capacity as a hospice nurse, I see dead people every working day. Well, sometimes they're not *all the way* dead, at times they're *almost* dead or they're *on the road to being dead fairly soon* but who isn't? Birth and death are two sides of the same coin and they're two of the most intimate actions a human being can witness. The only other act that compares in terms of intimacy is making love. Obviously I don't make love to my patients but it is a service of love that a hospice nurse renders. Patients and families I've just met become my closest friends in a matter of minutes.

They give me an all-access pass into their homes and their lives. They entrust me with the management of their death or the death of their loved one. It's an enormous responsibility and one I do not take lightly.

Under no circumstances can this be considered a *"how to die"* book, nor is it an instruction manual designed to teach the layperson how to care for a dying patient. It's a collection of true deaths that have touched my heart and my soul, and changed me. Dealing with patients and their families, or caregivers, as they go through the dying process can be rewarding, touching, tragic, frustrating, frightening, disgusting, enlightening, spiritual, chaotic, hysterically funny and all of the above at once. My work as a hospice nurse is never dull.

I've cared for incredibly wealthy patients living in isolated compounds with their own staff of private-duty nurses, and desperate, homeless people who travel along the road of death in the backseat of an old van parked at a strip mall. The end is the same. Movie stars and politicians have mothers, fathers, grandparents and aunts and uncles who use hospice services. Drug dealers have brothers who get cancer or suffer strokes. Criminals have mothers, too, and sometimes they die on hospice. I've cared for the family members of CIA agents, police officers and district attorneys and at the same time I've been the nurse assigned to patients dying in homes that have been converted into meth labs and grow-houses. Like I said, my job is never boring.

My role is to midwife every patient into the next world with as much grace and dignity as possible. I guess the most astonishing thing is I'm good at it. I no longer see my patients as a set of systems or think of them as a series of tasks to complete. They are real to me. I laugh with them, I cry with them. Their stories are written on my heart. I remember their names.

1: How We Die

The Fisherman

I ONLY MET Robert Smith once but his death made a lasting impression on me because he died so well. The day of his admission to hospice, he was already unconscious and had been for over twenty-four hours. However, even if someone is unresponsive and, as we say, actively dying, protocol requires that I complete a brief physical assessment. I feel it would be rude of me to touch a stranger without an introduction, so despite his closed eyes and irregular breathing, I introduced myself to Bob.

I lightly brushed his forearm with my fingertips and explained that I would be listening to his heart and lungs and taking his blood pressure. Not surprisingly, because this happens all the time, he roused himself and smiled, acknowledging my presence with a direct look into my eyes, a look that said, "I know exactly who you are, what you want and what you're doing. Get on with it." He deliberately winked at me before closing his eyes and drifting off into what I can only describe as a death-sleep.

A death-sleep is a kind of in-between state where the person is still attached to the body and cognizant of everything around him, but he or she may or may not respond. I like to imagine my patients adrift in a boat tethered to the body with a long rope. I always tell families that although their loved one appears to be unconscious, if he or she really needs to say something, he or she will wake up and say it. This is also the point in the dying process when things in the environment can most strongly affect the patient. For instance, if the room is crowded, if it's hot and noisy, if there's crying, screaming, breast-beating, wailing, or if for some reason the patient has not received enough pain medication, the person can have difficulty cutting that rope and moving on.

Bob was a fisherman who had inoperable, widely metastasized lung cancer. The cancer hadn't responded to any treatment and his doctors sent him home from the hospital with a hospice referral. Initially, he declined our assistance. He thought it might still be possible to beat this thing by sheer force of will if nothing else, but then he experienced an epiphany. He and his son took their boat out for a three-day fishing trip on the Sacramento Delta. According to Bob's son they had a great time, caught a lot of fish, drank a lot of beer and on the last day, Bob, in a quiet moment which is a rarity on the windy Delta, said, "I'm going to die, aren't I." His son told me Bob wasn't asking a question.

When they returned home, Bob called his family together and made it clear that he would be gone very soon. He, his wife and their three children sat around the kitchen table drinking coffee and they had the opportunity to say everything that needed to be said. Then Bob stopped eating and drinking and refused any medication. The next day he showered, brushed his teeth and put himself to bed. He very quickly sank into a semi-comatose state.

By the time I became involved in his care, three days later, the family was psychologically and emotionally prepared for his death and in fact, they were looking forward to it for his sake. It was very simple in their minds. Bob wanted to die without too much interference, and his family wanted to be with him. He'd given them very specific instructions—he did not want diapers and he refused a hospital bed.

His wife matter-of-factly informed me, "If he poops, we'll clean him up. If he needs to be turned, we'll turn him. He's instructed us that we are not to hover. We intend to follow his wishes."

Bob's family didn't need my help, not really. Like Bob they were a self-sufficient bunch, self-contained, strong and quietly confident. All I did was provide them with medication to keep Bob comfortable in the event that he needed it, and instructions for care that would ease his passing. The family didn't want any hand-holding. No hovering.

WHEN I WAS a kid growing up in Iowa, I used to fish every Saturday at Lake Manawa. It was an all-day kind of activity that required patience and the ability to stay still and be quiet for long periods. I had to learn not to fuss with the line. That is the waiting for death. Don't fuss with the line. Be patient and be still. Death will bite when it's good and ready. No hovering.

Bob died peacefully twelve hours after my visit. When he died, his son had been sitting quietly at his bedside reading a book. His wife and two daughters were asleep in the other room. He died the way he had lived, without a fuss and on his own terms.

I find that people usually do that, die the way they've lived. If their life was weird, their death can be even weirder. If family dynamics were negative, they don't usually improve as death approaches. As a matter of fact, any negativity typically gets worse and makes the death drawn out and difficult, and often fills the actual death scene with unnecessary drama.

I've found that some of my patients will attempt to

avoid a scene altogether by waiting until the watching family member steps out to "just get a cup of coffee" or "use the bathroom" and then they hurry and die before anyone can get back in the room. Sometimes I think my patients do that to spare everyone they love the pain of having to witness the actual death. Other times I think they see their opportunity to bolt and they get the hell out. Nothing is harder for me as a hospice nurse than to witness a patient take his last, peaceful breath, and as I prepare to pronounce him dead, a hysterical family member bursts into the room and hurls herself onto the dead body, dragging the soul back in with a terrible, rattling gasp. On rare occasions I've seen this push and pull last for hours, until the body can't take anymore and finally gives up the ghost. It's very tragic for everyone when this happens.

Death is far more than a mere physical process. There's a lot of other stuff going on, spiritual, emotional, and mental stuff, but unless you work with it on a daily basis, unless you make *death* your career, it's difficult, if not impossible to see beyond the obvious. The obvious being the loss of someone you love, or the loss of someone with whom you've at least had a relationship, good or bad.

There are two main pieces to the dying puzzle, the family and the patient. In Bob's case his family understood, without any input from me, how to let him go. But Bob accepted his role. He agreed with the process. He agreed to die. There was no pressing need for him to die right at that moment, he had a choice. Bob was relatively young and other than his lung cancer, reasonably healthy. He could have lasted several weeks to several months. He *chose* not to linger, my emphasis being on the word, *chose*. Sometimes my patients choose to die. Sometimes my patients do the exact opposite. They choose to outlive their own bodies. Unfortunately, they turn into what I've come to think of as *walking corpses.*

Mrs. Brown

TAKE MRS. BROWN, for instance. She became a walking corpse out of necessity. The matriarch of four generations, she lived with her daughter and her daughter's boyfriend, her two grandchildren and their significant others, and her two precocious great-grandchildren in an immaculately clean but crowded two bedroom, one bath condominium. Mrs. Brown had raised her daughter and her two grandchildren and at the time of her cancer diagnosis she was also responsible for rearing her two great-grandchildren. So many people depended upon her that she was unwilling to accept her terminal diagnosis. Although she agreed to hospice services to satisfy her daughter, it quickly became apparent to all of us involved in her case that she intended to live in the *Land of Denial* until the bitter end. I always say, a little denial can go a long way.

Mrs. Brown had advanced stomach cancer and her physician expected her to live two weeks at the most. She lasted four months post-discharge from the hospital. To describe her state of being as *alive* would be an exaggeration. Mrs. Brown seemed to mummify before our very eyes, yet she somehow miraculously continued to inhale and exhale and manage her household affairs in her utterly desiccated condition.

Sometimes I'd arrive at the crowded home for a scheduled visit, expecting to find her in bed, only to be guided to a small walk-in closet or the storage shed on the patio by the great-grandson. I'd find Mrs. Brown propped stiffly against a wall, frozen in the middle of some task, looking exactly like a log of wood set out to cure. She'd appear to have been dead for centuries, dehydrated in the sands of the Sahara, or freeze-dried in the snows of the Andes. Sometimes I feared that one touch from me and she'd crumble to dust. The experience shook me. I was both horrified and fascinated by her tenacity.

Mrs. Brown tried to avoid Death by clinging with desperation her usual tasks. Unfortunately she'd quickly become exhausted, lean against something to rest and stiffen in place. At one point the social worker and I were forced to carry Mrs. Brown out of a clothes closet. I took her upper body to protect her head, the social worker took her lower body and we literally carried her beneath our arms like a two by four. Under other circumstances, it would have been a comical scene instead of a tragedy.

When Mrs. Brown finally died her family didn't even realize she'd gone, and her body sat stiffly on a stool in the linen closet for four hours. I made the death call, or visit, and I genuinely understood their mistake. Her eyes were open and she looked exactly as she'd looked for months. To my great relief, the family opted for cremation because I was terrified Mrs. Brown would spring back to life during the embalming process. Unlike Bob, Mrs. Brown was definitely not ready to die and her spirit outlasted her physical body. She made a choice.

Thanks to Mrs. Brown, I learned not only to respect such determination, but I learned how to accept and care for patients like her on their own terms. I learned how to meet her very unique physical, emotional and spiritual needs.

Mrs. Brown didn't avoid death because she was afraid. She had no fear of death. She refused to die until she was certain her great-grandsons were taken care of. The very day of her death adoption papers came through for the boys and they were officially adopted by Mrs. Brown's daughter, their grandmother. That's what Mrs. Brown had been waiting for.

In my experience, it's extremely rare for patients to be afraid of death when it finally arrives, maybe before, if they have the time and the wherewithal to think about it but never when they die. As a matter of fact, I can only recall one patient in my entire nursing career, both in the hospital and with hospice, who was afraid up until the very instant of her death.

AS A NEW graduate working in Intensive Care, I received a *dump*. In other words, I was assigned a patient nobody knew what to do with. She was dying, nothing could change that. The family refused to take her home. In their defense a referral to hospice was not common at the time. However, they were unwilling to remain at her bedside. It fell to me to keep her company in her final hours. *Lucky her.*

I have to be honest. This was not my finest moment. I had two other patients to care for who were in critical condition and there were things I could do to help them. I could not help this woman. She was a direct admission from the emergency room and she had no doctor listed other than the on-call physician who had never seen her. I spoke with her family by phone and they made it crystal clear to me that they didn't want to be involved. They simply requested a call when she died. I had absolutely no medications ordered for her other than a very mild sedative/antihistamine.

I hadn't been working on the unit long and I wasn't sure how far I could push the on-call doctor. Back then, health care professionals weren't as into pain control as we are now. I'm pretty sure some physicians at that time were still insisting infants couldn't feel pain due to an immature nervous system and therefore didn't bother to medicate them before certain very painful procedures. I suspect very few nurses and doctors on duty that night gave more than a passing thought to my patient. Actually, I suspect everyone tried hard not to think about her. I, of course, didn't have that luxury.

It was clear to me as soon as I admitted her that I was

in for a long night. Within thirty minutes I realized I could not care for her along with my other two patients. Her violent struggle with death demanded all of my attention. Coworkers were willing to pick up my other patients, but they avoided this woman's room like the plague.

As I said, I do not remember the names of my patients from those days, but I remember her demographics as if it was yesterday. I can still read the information sheet like it's printed in my memory. She was five feet, seven inches tall and she weighed approximately one hundred and fifteen pounds. She was eighty-two years old and she'd been widowed for twenty-five years. She had a daughter living in town and a son living somewhere on the East Coast. I don't recall reading anything in the note about grandchildren. A neighbor hadn't seen her in several days and she became concerned. She contacted the patient's daughter. When her daughter unlocked the front door to check on her mother she found her breathing, but unresponsive, on the living room floor. The daughter called the paramedics. The patient opened her eyes once in the ambulance. The emergency room doctor diagnosed a severe cerebral vascular accident, or stroke, and her daughter requested, appropriately, that nothing be done.

By the time the patient was delivered to me, she was screaming at the top of her lungs and flailing her arms in every direction. As soon as we transferred her into a bed, everyone fled the room and left me alone with her. It's not as if the other nurses were cowards and I was the courageous Florence Nightingale, she was my patient, I couldn't leave the room.

I attempted to calm this woman by every means I could think of, that I had actual orders for and that common sense dictated, but I was unsuccessful. Nurses peeked into the room every few minutes or so and instructed me to keep her quiet for the sake of the other patients. It became increasingly clear to me that there was no way that was going to happen. This patient was doing battle with the Angel of Death.

As I said, I remember her stats but I had no clue what had transpired in her life. What caused her to experience such a terrible struggle? I didn't know if she'd been a good person, a bad person, or simply led a very difficult life. Did she have a whole lot of unfinished business? Was she toting major emotional baggage along with her?

Now, as a hospice nurse, I would recognize what we describe as severe end-stage agitation and I would have plenty of medications on hand to deal with her suffering. Back then, not only was I unsure as to what was happening, more significantly I didn't have anything available to help her.

What bothered me most was the terror in this woman's eyes. I couldn't see what she saw, but I could look into her eyes and I've never seen eyes so filled with fear in my life. She scared the bejeezus out of me. If the doctor had been willing to give me reasonable medication orders, I would have sedated her simply to help her close her eyes. All I had were orders for an antihistamine to be given intramuscularly. I gave her the maximum dose but of course it wasn't strong enough to make a dent.

She and I could just as easily have been in a boxing arena as in a hospital room. She was the boxer and I played the role of trainer. Her bed became her corner and when the bell sounded in her head she'd come out of her corner swinging. She punched, kicked and wrestled her way around the room, weaving and bobbing and shouting. Then I guess the bell would sound again to end the round, because she'd collapse into my arms and I'd haul her back into bed and unsuccessfully try to get her to stay there.

The worst part of it wasn't the fighting, it was the pointing. There was something in the corner, something I couldn't see. Her eyes would focus on it and open wide in horror. She'd point a long, bony finger at the corner, her mouth moving silently. She'd finally let out an ear-splitting shriek and jump out of bed to start the fight all over again.

Although I was unable to see what was in that corner, in my heart I believe the Angel of Death waited there and I don't think he resembled Brad Pitt. My hair stood on end whenever I was forced to dodge and weave my way past the back corner of the room. I tried to avoid looking in that direction but it was like passing a car accident on the freeway, you try not to rubberneck but you fail every time.

PATIENTS FREQUENTLY ASK me, how will it be, to die? Will I be scared? I always answer them as truthfully as I can, that it will be fine, everything will be okay. Nobody is ever afraid when they die. They might be afraid before, but never when they die. It's my guarantee, my promise to my hospice patients. When death comes they will not be afraid. This was true of my patients even when I worked Intensive Care, before I knew the first thing about hospice nursing. This particular patient, for whatever reason, was the one exception to that promise.

AFTER SEVEN HOURS, every muscle, every joint and every bone in my body ached. I was exhausted, she was still fighting. I took a chance and utilized Intensive Care *standing orders*. Because of new rules and regulations, *standing orders*, or emergency orders, no longer exist in most healthcare facilities. I used an order for a different medication. I intended to inject her with a strong muscle relaxant to see if that might succeed in calming her.

I discussed this with my nursing supervisor and she agreed wholeheartedly. So, very young and inexperienced but utterly determined, I marched to the locked med cart, unlocked it, drew up the medication under the watchful eye of my supervisor, relocked the med cart and returned to her room. As I entered, she bolted upright in bed, her trembling hand pointing to the corner, her mouth agape in a toothless scream. I wasn't having any of it. I was going to help her, by God. She would calm down and die peacefully. If it killed her, I was going to make this work.

"Mrs. Blank!" I yelled over her screams, "Mrs. Blank! I'm going to give you another shot. I promise you this one will help you relax. I promise."

She ignored me and continued to point at the corner, mouthing gibberish. I got a firm grip on her right thigh, picked a spot with some meat, cleansed a small area with an alcohol pad and shoved that needle in all the way to the hub.

Then it happened. Before I could even withdraw the plunger slightly to check for blood, her soul exploded out of that pinhole like air from a ruptured tire. I saw it. I felt it. An icy blast tore past me, blowing my hair straight back and whipping my baggy scrubs around my body. Frozen in horror, I watched a yellow ripple start at the site of the injection and flow up Mrs. Blank's body until it reached her head. Her mouth still open, her hand still pointing at the corner, she fell back on the pillow, dead. I proceeded to do the only thing that made any sense at that moment, scream my bloody head off!

The nursing staff came running. The Charge Nurse slammed the door shut behind her and clamped a hand over my mouth to stifle my screams. She tried to shush me, and when that failed, she reminded me that we had critical patients who could hear everything. With those words, I regained enough self-control to stop shrieking, but I continued to hyperventilate. She wrapped a strong arm around my waist and with a hand still over my mouth, dragged me down to the emergency room. Someone shoved a paper bag into my hands, but I was shaking too much to hold it to my mouth. The ER doctor held it for me.

He patted my back kindly as I attempted to slow my breathing and he asked, "What? You've never seen a patient die before?"

"No, that's not it," I croaked from inside the bag.

"Well what? Did she bleed out then? That can be very disturbing."

I shook my head. "No."

"Well, what is it then?" He asked, impatient now.

"It was the way she died. She died," I sobbed, "because I poked her with a hypodermic needle."

His response was a resounding, "Huh?"

I pulled the paper bag away from my mouth and told him the story. He was nice enough to listen without laughing and if he thought I was a lunatic, he kept it to himself.

Finally, he took my hand and said, "Look at it this way, you released her. She was obviously having trouble getting out and when you stuck her, you let her out. It's okay, you didn't do anything wrong." And with that, he gave my hand a final pat and went to meet an ambulance.

I sat alone in the ER cubicle, ignoring the chaos around me and contemplated his hypothesis. I came to the conclusion that even if he was merely trying to humor me, he'd hit the nail on the head. I poked a hole in her and let her out. I have no explanation for everything else that occurred but I will say this, since becoming a hospice nurse, I've been with a number of patients who have dramatically escaped their bodies when they were poked by a needle or otherwise prodded in some way. Sometimes it happens during a simple dressing change.

Home Health Aides in particular are well aware of the phenomenon and when they handle a patient very close to death they treat them like spun glass. I think it's happened at least once to everyone I've worked with. You turn a patient from one side to the other, they exhale loud and long, and they die. It's something I always keep in mind and I warn families when I think there's a need but I'm cautious because I find caregivers are then reluctant to turn the patient. It happened to one of my families just two weeks ago. Forewarned is forearmed, I guess. It's better to be prepared than to end up in the ER with a paper bag over your face.

ALL OF THE above brings me to the subject of *Death* itself. On one occasion I had a patient dying in a Skilled Nursing Facility, otherwise known as a nursing home. I managed her symptoms well with medication and positioning. She was dying very comfortably. As a matter of fact, her dying was textbook perfect. Her physician and I happened to be in the facility at the same time and we were both keeping a close eye on her. Her son was also present.

This *death business*, as he kept referring to it, made him extremely uneasy. Sometimes I think family members need sedation far more than my patients. He could not sit still. He paced back and forth at the patient's bedside, muttering, unable to sit in the nice soft chair I found for him. He was driving me a bit nuts so I left the room and headed to the nurse's Station. Fortunately for his dying mother, unfortunately for me, he trailed after me. All the way down the hall he kept repeating, "But why? But why?" There wasn't a single answer I could give him that he found satisfactory. I found myself increasingly frustrated, not with his mother, she was doing just fine, but with him and with my own inability to answer his questions in a way he could comprehend.

The doctor happened to be sitting at the nurse's Station. I pulled up a chair next to her and buried my face in the patient's chart, hoping to discourage the son from his constant questioning. He started in on the doctor with his *but whys*. The doctor, in typical doctor fashion, launched into a long-winded and very technical explanation of what transpires during the dying process. She proceeded to very specifically list all his mother's many illnesses and how each and every one of them contributed to her dying. I could tell by the look on the poor man's face that he was growing more confused and anxious with each word the doctor spoke.

He finally blurted out, "But what's killing her? What?" The doctor turned to me in a mute appeal for help.

I looked the man straight in the eyes and told him flatly and in no uncertain terms, "Death. Death is killing your mother."

He stood there for a second, a stunned expression on his face, and then he replied, "Ooooohhhh," and he meandered back down the hallway.

The doctor crooked an eyebrow and gave me a funny look but she didn't say anything more.

When next I looked in on his mother, I found the son in the soft chair, half-asleep, a hand resting on his mother's arm. She died peacefully minutes later. It was a good death and I stayed with her son until the body was removed by the mortuary and he left the facility. He coped remarkably well once his question was answered.

Isn't that *the* question: But why? Hasn't that always been the great existential question man has asked throughout history? Or one of the two questions man has asked since he became self-aware? The first question being what is the meaning of life, and the second, a two-parter, why do we die and what happens after death? I can answer with certainty the first part of that two-part question. Hospice patients die from lots of things, but in the end it all comes down to just *one* thing, Death. They all die from Death.

2: Oh the First Days
Are the Hardest Days

John

ALTHOUGH I'VE HAD many favorite patients, John tops my list. Possibly because he was my first official hospice patient, maybe because he reminded me of my grandfather who I dearly loved, maybe because he was just a plain old good guy and he died with such grace and dignity. I don't know for certain, but I do know that his death was very personal. As a matter of fact, his death was the first in a series of deaths that were all very personal, all patients I had grown quite attached to. Caring for them and watching them die really hit me hard. Their deaths reminded me of the innate unfairness of life, how bad things happen in what should be the best of times. I also learned during these few months early in my career that if my patients and their families can go through everything dying entails then I can help them through the process. Especially during those moments when instinct tells me to run the other way as fast as my legs can carry me.

John had widely metastasized lung cancer. He'd just finished radiation and he'd had a feeding tube inserted directly into his stomach because during his treatment, the radiation had gradually destroyed his ability to swallow. Despite that fact, he was actually doing well, up in his recliner most of the day, able to walk slowly around the neighborhood and meet with his friends on the corner for a daily gossip session. John never complained of pain. Frankly, he never complained about anything.

Visiting him was a pleasure for me. He and his family accepted me as one of their own. We talked about medications and pain and bowels and all the usual hospice stuff, but only because we had to. Most of our conversations revolved around John's life. He spent a lot of time reflecting about his past, present and future, and talking about what gave him pleasure now that he was physically and temporally limited.

He'd tell me about how much he relished a good steak. He'd chew it, suck all the flavorful juices out of the piece of meat then spit it out since he couldn't swallow. He loved his daily walks with his son. He was devoted to his indoor and outdoor cats, his backgammon games and his music. He loved jazz and an old Big Band album was usually playing when I arrived for a visit.

In my experience, lung cancer progresses something like this: Cancer. Treatment. Cancer. Treatment. Cancer. Treatment. Cancer. No more available treatment. Plateau. Plateau. Plateau. Pain crisis. Rapid Decline. Death.

I don't know why this particular cancer progresses in this fashion, but every lung cancer patient I've ever cared for, unless they are already in the rapid decline stage by the time I admit them to hospice, follows this pattern. Since hospice patients rarely, if ever, have autopsies we don't know for sure, but I'm guessing that at some point the cancer reaches a critical mass and breaks something or breaks into somewhere, hence the pain crisis and the rapid decline

John was fortunate to have several months of relative stability.

One afternoon I arrived while our music therapist was with John, playing guitar and singing. John's recliner faced away from the door so I walked around it and a single glance at his face told me he had turned the corner and we were on the downhill side of life. My breath caught in my throat. His eyes were closed and a small smile played on his lips as he listened to the guitar but there were lines in his face that hadn't been there the day before. I saw something else. The ephemeral, transparent, sort of luminous quality to his skin I've come to recognize as approaching death told me he had mere days.

After the music therapist finished and packed up, I slipped my hand into his and he whispered, "Heidi, I'm in pain."

"Oh God . . ." I wanted to sob. "Not John." But I couldn't cry. I needed to fix his pain and I needed to be a steady ship to see him through to the end of his voyage. John's wife and I put John to bed and he never got out again. He lived four days. I saw him at least twice a day, keeping him as comfortable as possible and assisting his family with his care.

·When I arrived on the fourth day, John's wife greeted me at the door with the words, "He's asking for you."

Although he was no longer able to open his eyes, John could whisper and make his needs known. I went into the bedroom and took his hand. John smiled the sweetest smile. He knew he would die that day. He asked his family to leave the room and close the door. He didn't want them to witness his death. He preferred to spare them that memory. He just wanted me. I climbed onto the bed and put my arm around him, resting his head in the hollow of my shoulder. I rocked him like a baby until he died an hour later.

WHEN A GENTLE soul like John's leaves the body, it feels as if a breeze ruffles your hair. You sense a brief shift in shadow and light. You catch the faint scent of cloves. There's nothing concrete, nothing you can put your finger on. John left with a slow, smooth exhale.

My heart felt as heavy as a lead weight in my chest, but I couldn't allow myself to pay it any attention because it was my duty to smooth John's hair, position him peacefully on his pillows, open the door and tell the family he was gone.

Hysteria is not in my official job description though I am occasionally prone to it in my off hours. Families fall apart well enough on their own so it's up to me, as the hospice nurse, to keep it together and comfort them. It's very simple, someone has to remain calm and in these situations that would be me.

All that afternoon I sensed John right behind me, propping me up whenever I faltered, so I could do what needed to be done for him and for his family. His powerful presence helped me get through the agony of his death. Just the simple act of writing these words brings on the tears I couldn't shed that day. Sometimes I drive past his house and I see his outdoor cats sitting on the porch swing, looking like they're waiting for him to come around the block. I know I am

WHEN I WAS six years old, my grandfather fell sick with an unexplained illness. A year later, after a great many unpleasant tests, he was diagnosed with ALS, or Amyotrophic Lateral Sclerosis, also known as Lou Gehrig's Disease. ALS is a progressive neurological disorder that gradually strips you of your ability to walk, talk, feed yourself, swallow and eventually, breathe. There is no cure.

Most people with the disease die within four years.

Rarely, men like Stephen Hawking, the world renowned physicist, survive for a long time, completely dependent upon a great many caregivers and usually a portable ventilator. Despite the fact that we were children, my parents didn't spare us the details and my father explained very clearly why it was called Lou Gehrig's Disease. He said one of the greatest baseball players in the world, Lou Gehrig, died of ALS.

Every Saturday, my mother dropped me off at the public library. Being an avid reader even at that age, I walked up to Mildred Smock, the librarian, and asked for books about Lou Gehrig, the great baseball player. Miss Smock initially steered me into the Children's Room where I found several easy to read biographies about his years with the Yankees. I knew what the Yankees were because my grandmother performed in the local theatre and she'd done costume design for the play, *Damn Yankees*. She'd made sure we had front row seats. I was aware the Yankees were a perennially winning baseball team that had quite possibly sold their souls to the devil, at least according to the play.

In the children's books I was able to read all about Lou Gehrig's baseball career but nowhere did the books mention Lou Gehrig's Disease, so I returned to the information desk and requested an adult biography. That may sound like an odd thing for a seven-year-old kid to do, but I'd been reading since I was three and Mildred Smock was quite familiar with my idiosyncrasies.

"Follow me," she said.

We headed down the aisles toward the Biography Section and she pulled out a hardback book and handed it to me. I checked it out and read it from cover to cover. Thus, alongside the heartbreak I felt for my grandfather and the inevitable path this disease would take, was born my life-long admiration for Lou Gehrig. After all, he traveled the same road. He faced the disease with tremendous courage and he did it at the peak of his career. I've since seen film footage of his speech, July 4th, 1939, where in front of thousands of people, knowing he was going to die, he said he considered himself the luckiest man on the face of the earth. I've seen the movie version of his life too, *The Pride of the Yankees*. His character is played by Gary Cooper.

In both the real film footage and the movie, the speech never fails to move me to tears, for Lou Gehrig, for my grandfather and for every person who has died of the disease. It's not that dying of ALS is particularly painful, it's that ALS strikes the most active and engaged people and they simply fade away. It's not fair.

My grandfather lived two years after his diagnosis. He was lucky in that he continued to walk, although he lost his voice and the strength in his hands quite early. Several days before his death, I remember riding with my mom over to the VA hospital in Omaha, Nebraska, where my grandfather had been admitted for some tests. He wanted to come home for just a little while. I think he knew his death was approaching.

I waited with him while my mom went to check him out of the hospital. He sat on the edge of his bed and slowly leaned over to slip on his shoes. He used a long shoehorn to slide them over his heels as his hands were very weak. I zipped up his jacket for him. He nodded at me and patted my head. We sat side by side on the hospital bed, waiting. I promised myself I would not cry because I didn't want to make him cry, so I just leaned against him. I desperately wanted to feel him before he was gone forever.

At that time in my life my grandfather was the most important person in the world to me. He loved me and I adored him. He had a great many talents but he'd never amounted to much and he was certainly not a financial success. But he was a kind and gentle man who lovingly raised

four children. His children had given him twelve grandchildren who meant everything to him. My grandfather was
nothing special to the world but he was special to me. He
was just a regular guy doing the best he could. I liked to
think of Lou Gehrig the same way. Just a regular guy doing
the best he could, like my grandfather, like John.

After my mother finished with the checkout process,
she came to get us. My grandfather shuffled down the long
corridor to the exit. I don't think my mom was very comfortable with this process because I was the one who remained glued to his side in case he stumbled. My mom and
I were silent on the drive home, while my grandfather listened to a baseball game on the car radio. He stayed with
us for the weekend.

On Sunday, he made it known to my parents that he
wanted to return to the hospital. I didn't go along this time.
He turned and looked into my eyes just before he walked
out the front door. I saw a little sadness, but more than that
I saw detachment and resignation and I knew with absolute
certainty I'd never see him again. I thought my heart might
stop beating then and there. I ran upstairs, threw myself on
my bed and cried myself to sleep. My parents stayed with
him at the hospital. He stopped breathing that night and
died peacefully. My parents gave us the news the next
morning.

Death doesn't seems real when it happens to someone
you love. I learned it then and I relearned it working with
John. For years, I waited for my grandfather to come back.
I believed that one day the door would open and he'd be
standing there with open arms, smiling at me, calling for his
bunchke, his nickname for me. I'd exclaim, *Zaida*, my Yid-
dish version of grampa, and I'd ask him, *where have you been?*

I'd imagined that I'd come running and jump into his
arms. I'd rub my face against his scratchy wool button-
down shirt like I always did, and he'd pull a handful of

penny candy out of his jacket pocket and dump it into my open hands like he always did. My parents wondered why I never cried at the funeral. I couldn't. I can't. I loved him too deeply. Like John's cats, I'm still waiting for him to come around again.

Mara

A FEW WEEKS after John's death, I lost another patient I'd grown very fond of. Her diagnosis was also lung cancer. On the surface, Mara seemed like a tough old broad who just wanted to be left alone. She rebuffed almost every attempt her family made to help her. However, beneath her hard-as-nails exterior was a brilliant woman with a remarkable past. I spent hours listening to her stories. Besides, I'm partial to cranky old ladies. Mara would push you away just to see how far you'd go. If you came back unafraid, you'd passed her test and she'd let you into her life.

Honestly, I didn't just like Mara, I loved her. She and I could talk about everything. Nothing was taboo between us, men, sex, fashion, food and recipes, wine, music, books, pets we'd loved and lost, families and surprisingly enough, World War II. I learned after Mara's death that she'd been a spy for the United States government in the 1940's.

As far as I can make out, Mara and her husband were stationed in London early in the War. Both were fluent in French and German, and after the Nazis occupied Paris, they traveled there. If I remember correctly, her husband's cover was that of a wealthy investor, a Nazi sympathizer interested in German manufacturing. He was accompanied, of course, by his very beautiful and intriguing blonde wife. She literally charmed the information she wanted out of the German elite.

Mara's daughter showed me photos taken at cocktail parties in occupied Paris. They were something straight out of a Nazi propaganda film. Mara looked just like Greta

Garbo, she even held her cigarette like her, which explains, of course, the lung cancer. Apparently, Mara and her husband would pass the information they gathered, in code, to the Allies. Her daughter, Betty, actually found a wrapped, yellowed bundle of coded messages after her death, not that she could decipher any of them. Had Mara and her husband been captured, they'd most certainly have been either executed or sent to a Concentration Camp.

As our relationship progressed, Mara became like a grandmother to me. Her daughter and I alternated days so that one of us could make her lunch and serve it to her. Stubborn as she was, Mara refused to admit that she could no longer prepare meals for herself. Most days she was too short of breath to walk into the kitchen. Her daughter and I played along. One of us would just happen to show up at noon and remark, "Oh, by the way, I'm hungry. How about I make us a little something?"

I'd carry lunch into the living room on a tray and literally sit at her feet as she ate and regaled me with tales of her colorful life. Of course that gave me an opportunity to tidy the kitchen and bathroom, make the bed, check her meds on the sly and set up dinner.

One subject and one subject only remained off-limits, cancer. Mara made it clear from the beginning that I was not to utter the word. So I never did. Not even when I arrived one day and found her clutching her chest, unable to catch her breath and suffering excruciating pain. One glance told me that the largest tumor, which had wrapped itself around her heart, had very likely eroded into a ventricle or was putting too much pressure on her cardiac muscle and she was probably suffering a heart attack.

I began hyperventilating and my natural impulse was to run for the phone and dial 9-1-1. Then my forebrain kicked in and I stopped mid-stride. I remembered, *oh yeah, I'm a hospice nurse. She's a DNR, Do Not Resuscitate. She's sup-*

posed to die. She doesn't want me to call 9-1-1. She doesn't want to go to the hospital. Just to be on the safe side, I asked Mara if she wanted me to call the paramedics. She shook her head and mouthed the word, "No."

With one hand I made a call to her daughter and with the other, I started squirting liquid morphine into her mouth. From my days in Coronary Care, I was very comfortable with the use of morphine for heart attacks and I had to get her pain under control as quickly as possible. I knew Mara was in bad shape because for once she didn't argue with me. I no longer remember how many outrageous milligrams of the drug she required to take just the edge off her pain.

By the time her daughter arrived, Mara was resting on her daybed, but this was just the opening salvo. For the next week, 24/7, her daughter and I fought the Battle of the Bulge over and over again, trying desperately to stay ahead of Mara's pain. Unfortunately we lost the battle. It wasn't until the very last day of her life that Mara was finally comfortable enough to let go and die.

All of us involved in Mara's care were so exhausted by the time it was over that we could barely speak. We sank to the floor on whatever side of the hospital bed we happened to be on and gazed around the now peaceful room that had, up until a moment ago, been our battlefield. It was littered with the detritus of death: diapers and pads, used tissues, cut-up tee-shirts, sheets, towels and wet wash cloths, damp pillowcases, mouth swabs, alcohol wipes, lotion, garbage bags, bottles of morphine and lorazepam, a sedative, in various concentrations and stages of emptiness, suppository wrappers, pizza boxes and Chinese take-out.

Betty looked over at me, her beautiful face so like her mother's, now drawn and pale. She managed a wan smile and said, "It's what she wanted but if I'd known it was going to be like . . ." and she broke down.

I crawled to her, pushing aside the mess. A great battle had taken place. We huddled together on the bloody field, clinging to each other, the only two survivors.

Betty and I kept in touch for years and last I spoke with her, she mentioned that she still feels guilty. She wonders if there was anything more she could have done to help her mother in that final week. There was nothing more she could have done. She did everything right and her mother died in her own home, just as she wanted.

I remind Betty that families often second-guess themselves. They frequently wonder if there was one more thing they could have done, one more thing they should have said. I try to prepare families for this. It's not always easy to die. It's never easy to watch. I tell family members up front that caring for a loved one as they die is the hardest thing they will ever do. Hospice is available for support and symptom management, but the bulk of the care typically falls to family members and friends.

It's a lot easier on the dying person. They can be in familiar surroundings. They are free to interact with their loved ones and even with their pets. Nobody is sticking an IV into them, drawing blood, taking vital signs, waking them for pills, or in general, doing things that make them miserable. Once you're on hospice, at least if you're my patient, you can eat whatever you want, drink whatever you want, do whatever you want within reason, visit with whomever you want, or not. I'm a pushover. I don't insist my patients take any medicine they don't want to take.

My patients make their own decisions. Unless they can't make decisions and then I try to respect the family's wishes as much as possible.

Betty's persistent feelings of guilt are atypical. More often, families are flooded with immediate feelings of relief and gratitude. Relief because their loved one is no longer suffering and gratitude because they were able to spend those final days, weeks or months with them. Then come sadness and a sense of loss, though usually, with time, the memories of death are replaced with memories of life and whatever initial guilt a family member may feel, dissipates.

A little over a year ago, Betty left her job and since I no longer have her home phone number, I lost contact with her. Not a day goes by that I don't think of her and her mother. In case she's reading this book, I just want her to know.

Jeanine

JEANINE AND MARA lived two blocks apart. Since they were on my case load at the same time, I'd usually park between the two houses and walk from one to the other. They died two weeks apart.

Jeanine was an amazing woman. In her early sixties, she could be best described as a dynamo, youthful, bright, articulate, optimistic, uncomplaining in the extreme and, merely by an unpleasant quirk of fate, dying of pancreatic cancer. She'd just returned from an extended trip to the British Isles for one last pilgrimage to her favorite historic sites and on the advice of her oncologist, she accepted hospice.

She was mine, all mine. I refused to share Jeanine with anyone and the one and only time she saw a different nurse during my vacation, I returned to find her furious because that nurse wanted to talk about things like constipation and medications and pain and death. When the nurse arrived for a second visit, Jeanine shoved her out the door and slammed it in her face. She and I never talked about that stuff. Jeanine made it clear during our very first meeting that she would die on her own terms. That meant using medications when and only when she needed them, continuing her routine activities, living independently although she had a daughter nearby who was more than willing to help out, and when the time came, dying in the hospital surrounded by her friends from the cancer center. Regardless of what anyone else in my office thought about the situation, I had no problem accepting her conditions. Her sovereign wishes were my commands.

Jeanine was one of the lucky ones. The symptoms of pancreatic cancer are vague and many people tend to ignore them. In my experience, most patients with pancreatic cancer are dead within a month of their diagnosis. Because her late husband had been in the military, Jeanine was able to enroll in a government-sponsored experimental cancer program and she lived five full healthy years after treatment before her cancer recurred. Even once she was on hospice, Jeanine remained surprisingly well. She had occasional episodes of nausea and vomiting, but we found multiple medications that were effective and in the four and a half months I knew her, she never let a little inconvenient nausea slow her down.

Jeanine was a real gourmand and she loved to eat out. She told me that sometimes she'd feel queasy in the middle of dinner, excuse herself, vomit in the lady's room, and then return to the table to finish her meal. Her *bulimia* stories kept us both amused. She loved to use her cancer as a backdoor entry into exclusive restaurants all over the Bay Area. She told me she wanted to eat in the best before she died. Only one very well-known restaurant refused her and their attitude made her furious.

She exclaimed angrily, "Even telling them I was dying didn't do the trick! Can you believe it! That never fails!"

Her son, a multi-millionaire businessman visited that weekend and she enlisted his aid, but he couldn't get a table either. Jeanine may be dead and gone but I still haven't forgiven the place, because I know very well the manager saves tables for last minute celebrity guests.

A wonderful local chef graciously made room for

Jeanine and her son at the last minute and he personally served them a glorious meal. Jeanine called it surf and turf. I think the chef included crab, lobster, scallops and a filet mignon, not to mention the à la carte side dishes he provided. I know firsthand how incredible the place is. When she described the meal, Jeanine gleefully reported to me that she only threw up once. She was thrilled. Unfortunately, the outing to the restaurant was her last big hurrah.

Jeanine and I had made a pact. She promised to keep me apprised of her decline and I promised to tell her honestly when her death was no more than a week away. We'd built a lot of trust between us and I'm pretty good at making that kind of prediction. The only problem was that we both dreaded the moment when one of us would have to speak up. However, the day finally arrived, and neither of us could deny the facts.

I visited one morning and found Jeanine unable to get out of bed. She'd never suffered any pain during her entire illness, but that morning her nausea was quite severe and I couldn't settle her stomach with the many meds we had available. I took a good, hard look at her, sat at her bedside and we had the unavoidable conversation.

Jeanine was feeling pretty puny but her mind was clear and she accepted what I had to say with aplomb. I offered to call her daughter. She knew as well as I did that her daughter would willingly stay with her in her own home until the end, but Jeanine refused. She couldn't bear the thought of being totally dependent on a family member.

Jeanine confided to me just how much her home meant to her. Most people I work with prefer to die in familiar surroundings, but Jeanine said she absolutely couldn't die in her home. She told me it would be too hard to let go. So I confirmed the arrangements with the cancer center where she'd received the experimental treatment. They'd been expecting my call for months and were prepared to wave the red tape. Then I contacted Jeanine's daughter.

Jeanine issued instructions from the bed, her still shapely body racked by frequent spasms, as I packed her favorite nightgowns, socks, underwear and toiletries. I was struck by the eerie similarities between this experience with Jeanine and the experiences I'd had with women in labor at home when we packed for an unintended trip to the hospital.

The entire scene felt surreal and I moved through the house in a daze. I wasn't sending Jeanine to a happy ending. She wouldn't be returning home with a bundle of joy in her arms. I was sending my new best friend off to die. What a strange thing to do.

At last I bagged up the medications in case Jeanine needed anything during the forty-minute drive, grabbed her purse and her favorite pillows and opened the screen door for her daughter. This was the first time I'd met her and she was just like her mom, beautiful, strong, intelligent and determined to hold herself together as long as necessary.

Between the two of us, we got Jeanine and her bags into the car. I reclined her seat, fastened her seatbelt, tucked her pillows securely around her, showed her where I'd stashed her medications in her purse, handed her a plastic basin in case of an emergency, and placed a can of cold ginger ale in the nearest cup holder.

Weak as a newborn kitten, Jeanine leaned out the open car door to give me a kiss then handed me her house keys. We had agreed in advance that I would lock up the house and transport her cat to her daughter's home. I said goodbye and shut the car door as softly as I could. I waited at the curb as they pulled away, watched them turn around at the end of the block and waved as they passed me again, waved goodbye with a smile on my face as if Jeanine was leaving on vacation.

I stood at the curb until the car disappeared from view and then wandered back into the house and plopped down on Jeanine's lavender-colored sofa. I completely lost track of time in the empty house. Finally, Jeanine's white cat hopped into my lap and reminded me why I was still there. I buried my face in her long, thick hair and sobbed. She was willing to put up with this display of emotion for only a few minutes before she'd had enough and she began to meow for food. Obviously Jeanine hadn't fed her that morning. I should have realized. I rummaged through the cupboards until I found the bag of cat food and filled her dish. While I waited for the cat to eat, I explored. The house seemed far too quiet and the quiet made me uncomfortable. I required some tangible reminder of Jeanine's warm presence. I wanted to hear her infectious laugh, to feel alive in her space.

I understood Jeanine's love for the cozy home. Jeanine had decorated it in various shades of purple, the color of royalty, with lavender flowers and violet motifs everywhere. She loved violets, lavender and Johnny-jump-ups. The flowers in her garden showed through the kitchen windows. Those she'd cut and arranged in vases on her counter the previous day surrounded me with color and sweet perfume.

Everything my gaze fell on bore Jeanine's stamp, her touch, her spirit.

I sank into the flowered cushions of the easy chair and my eyes roamed over the scattered displays of souvenirs she'd picked up on her travels to Great Britain. Jeanine and I shared an obsession with Tudor and Stuart England. We could argue for hours about which of us had been Anne Boleyn or her daughter, Elizabeth, in a past life. We passionately discussed details of the lives of the ancient kings and queens of Britain. I had never before met anyone who shared my interest to such a degree.

We whiled away entire afternoons gossiping about Henry VIII and his marital foibles, Edward Plantagenet and the War of the Roses, Geoffrey of Anjou and Matilda, Eleanor of Aquitaine and Henry II and their many children. We discussed the fact that history had given King John, of Robin Hood fame, a bad rap while remembering his brother, the absent crusader, King Richard the Lionhearted, with undue fondness.

A secret sisterhood grew between us in the months before Jeanine's death and I was reluctant to give our friendship up, to give her up. Nobody I'd ever met shared my passion like Jeanine, no one. Putting her into that car and watching her drive off to her death was one of the most difficult things I had ever done. The act seemed surreal.

Eventually, I caught the cat, coaxed her into her carrier and loaded her and her kitty supplies into my car. I turned back to lock the front door and found myself frozen on the porch. My hand refused to move. I couldn't bring myself to close the door, to close the door on Jeanine's life. I had to run back into the house and remember her as hard as I could, burn everything about her, every conversation, every laugh we'd shared, every cup of tea we drank together, into my memory. I think I walked through the house ten more times, picking up Jeanine's things at random and setting them down again before I forced myself to step outside and lock that door. Regardless of what I wanted, Jeanine was not coming back. Her absence left a big empty space in my heart.

I phoned Jeanine's daughter for daily updates. She said that while her mom was comforted to be with her friends at the cancer center, she was frustrated as hell to find death so elusive. She was sick of the nausea. Jeanine lasted five days on intravenous anti-emetics, anti-nausea medications, and stubborn woman that she was, remained awake until the very end.

Three months later, I answered my door. The mailman handed me a cardboard tube and my eyes opened wide. I was astonished because I spotted Jeanine's purple return address label stuck to it. When I saw the label, my hands started to shake. I grabbed the tube and ran for my sharpest paring knife. Carefully rolled up inside was a worn poster depicting all the kings and queens of Britain, from earliest recorded history to modern day. It was the poster Jeanine and I had referred to in our friendly discussions about the good king, the weak link, the product of the worst inbreeding, who suffered from insanity, who was a saint, which queens were the power behind the throne. I was overcome. From the grave Jeanine remembered me.

I framed the poster and it hangs at the foot of my bed, despite my husband's objection that it's just an old poster. For several years, I kept the cardboard tube in which it was packed on the bookcase in my bedroom. I smiled whenever my eye caught the return address label. Unfortunately, it disappeared during a remodel. When we unpacked everything we'd packed up, the tube was missing. I was devastated. It felt as if I'd lost Jeanine all over again. But as the unicorn said in the book *The Last Unicorn*, "I remember you." I remember Jeanine very well.

TWO SUMMERS AGO, my daughters and I followed in Jeanine's footsteps and made a pilgrimage to England. The first place we stopped was Westminster Abbey, where I cried over the marble effigies of the kings and queens, including those of both Elizabeth and her half-sister and nemesis, Mary. Our second and more meaningful visit was to The Tower of London which is not a tower at all but rather a collection of dwellings and fortifications begun by the earliest Norman kings, the oldest structure being the White Tower in the center of the enclosure. It has been the official dwelling of the kings and queens of England since William the Conqueror ruled in the Eleventh Century.

Nearly overcome with emotion, I stood on the royal execution ground, the very spot where Anne Boleyn lost her head to the executioner's sword, both executioner and sword imported from France. Our *Beefeater* tour guide was gracious enough to allow me to spend time alone in the Chapel of St. Peter ad Vincula, where both Anne and her poor cousin Katherine Howard, Henry's seventh wife, also beheaded, are buried. Access to both crypts is restricted and the area around the altar is roped off, but standing on my tip-toes, I could just make out the inscriptions over the burial sites.

Jeanine warned me the experience would be overwhelming and she was right, as usual. In another life, she would have been there with me. As a matter of fact, I suspect she was.

Jeanine's daughter didn't send the poster. To this day, I have no idea who did.

He Loves Me, He Loves Me Not

ELLEN SUFFERED A massive stroke. The paramedics, as they are wont to do, managed to revive her. Unfortunately, she had sustained severe brain damage and remained in a comatose state. Though Ellen could open her eyes, she merely stared vacantly at the ceiling. The doctors offered to insert a feeding tube into Ellen's stomach, but they couldn't offer Ellen's husband any hope. Ellen continued to waste away despite the feeding tube. Her husband's efforts to elicit any response from her failed and after months of trying, he finally asked her doctor to make a hospice referral. I'm so grateful she was assigned to me. Ellen was a gift.

Every moment I spent with this family was pure joy. Ellen and her husband lived in a mobile home. Quarters were cramped when Ellen, her husband, their two daughters and their husbands, all the grandchildren and Ellen's sister and brother-in-law were in residence, but nobody minded, least of all Ellen. The house was filled with love. Everyone contributed to her care.

Ellen had been beautiful when she was young and she remained beautiful throughout the dying process. Of course her family felt tremendous sadness and many tears were shed during the month I spent with them, but I never heard a single whine of self-pity from anyone. Ellen's daughters helped create a peaceful space for her. They burned scented candles and massaged her with her favorite lotions. Her husband affixed shelves to the wall above her bed and covered them with photos of happy times. Her grandchildren played board games on the floor near her bed, while her two cats snuggled against her sides and no-body worried about whether they'd be asked to *keep it down* or *go outside*.

Ellen and her husband met in high school. According to him, it was love at first sight. In fifty years of marriage, other than his period of service in World War II, they had never been apart. In rare quiet moments when it was just the two of us, he told me the pain of losing her was so se-vere it felt like he was being ripped in half. In the same breath, he said he'd always feel her love for him and he knew her love would keep him whole.

When Ellen died, we were all present, surrounding her bed, holding hands. For the briefest moment we were bathed in white light, as if the sun shone down on us through the roof, which was of course, impossible. Then, in the space of a heartbeat, she was gone.

The family members held each other quietly and every person gave me a warm hug. They invited me to spend the afternoon and we squeezed into the tiny kitchen where someone handed me a mug of hot chocolate. Someone else passed around a plate of warm, just-baked oatmeal-raisin cookies. While we waited for the mortuary staff to arrive, the family shared stories and celebrated Ellen's life as she lay dead not ten feet away from us. I swear I saw a smile form on her lips. I remember thinking as I leaned against the kitchen wall, it's times like these when we are truly tested.

Ellen's family passed their test with flying colors. I wish I could say the same for the Brady family, or for me.

MR. BRADY WANTED his wife Catherine to die at home. At least, that's what I was told. Catherine's ovarian cancer was widespread. It had invaded her entire abdominal cavity. Her surgeon opened her one last time to see if there was anything he could do to help. It only took him one quick look to decide to close her up again. There was nothing anyone could do.

Catherine suffered such severe cancer-related pain that she at first refused admission to hospice. She asked that she be allowed to die in the hospital, where her pain was under control and the nurses were managing her multiple medical and surgical problems very competently. Her doctor agreed to keep her as an inpatient and he ordered comfort care only.

Our Hospice Nurse Liaison heard about Catherine's case. It is the job of the Hospice Nurse Liaison to assist hospitals with patient discharges and to recruit appropriate patients for hospice. After all, hospice isn't merely a service, it's a business and businesses need customers. Cold though it may sound, people with a terminal illness are our customers.

The Hospice Nurse Liaison initiated multiple discussions with Catherine's husband and then with Catherine, and she finally convinced Mr. Brady he could bring Catherine home with complete confidence in hospice. She assured him we would take care of *anything* that came up. Assuming, from what they'd been told by our Nurse Liaison, that Catherine only had a few days left, her husband made the decision to bring her home and Catherine very reluctantly agreed.

Unaware of the extent of Catherine's medical needs and completely unprepared for the family issues I encountered, I met the ambulance at the Brady's beautiful, heavily wooded estate. The paramedics and I, following an impatiently gesturing Mr. Brady, gently lifted Catherine's gurney up and down several flights of stairs in their multi-level home until we came at last to a tastefully decorated sunroom where the hospital bed was already set up.

While I was still in the midst of transferring Catherine to the hospital bed, before I could utter a single word about signing hospice consents, Mr. Brady informed me brusquely, "How long is this going to take? I'm fifteen minutes late for a meeting."

"But Mr. Brady," I exclaimed, "you can't leave Mrs. Brady alone!"

"What the hell do you mean I can't leave her alone? I'm a busy man. You take care of her! That's your job, isn't it?" And with that statement, he turned on his heel and strode out of the room.

I chased after him only to have him slam the door of his Cadillac in my face and peel out of the driveway.

Shaking with distress and anger, I returned to the sunroom. One of the paramedics shot me a sympathetic look, but they had to leave. I tried to compose myself. Catherine, who unfortunately remained alert and oriented throughout her ordeal, gave me an understanding smile and whispered, "I'm sorry."

With my help to steady her hand, Catherine signed her own hospice consents.

Later that afternoon when I returned to the office, I discretely cornered the Nurse Liaison and asked her exactly what she had told the family. She initially tried to avoid answering my question, but I persisted. I voiced my concerns about the complicated nature of Catherine's case. I told her in all honesty, that Catherine's husband didn't seem to want her at home. He certainly didn't appear to understand the role of hospice and his own role in caring for his wife.

I stated that Catherine was very frightened at the prospect of dying at home and I questioned the appropriateness of the referral. With an apologetic shrug, the Nurse Liaison assured me that Catherine only had a few more days to live, so we could handle it. I wondered aloud how she came to that conclusion as the assessment I'd done on Catherine that morning clearly indicated otherwise. I said barring sepsis, Catherine could live several weeks. The Nurse Liaison merely repeated that in her opinion Catherine only had a few days to live, so I could deal with it. I wasn't concerned about whether or not *I* could deal with it and I respectfully repeated my doubts to her and to my supervisor about the feasibility of managing this case at home. My concerns fell on deaf ears.

Over the next two weeks, Catherine bravely attempted to manage her own medical care from her hospital bed, despite the fact that she could barely move. Those of us working on her case provided her with as much assistance as possible. Instead of passing away comfortably and quietly in the hospital where she could rely upon the staff nurses to provide her care, Catherine lingered. Her husband absolutely refused to participate. Her adult children never offered to come home, despite my phone calls outlining their mother's desperate situation. Shrugging off my offer to help arrange for twenty-four hour hired care, Mr. Brady said he didn't want *a stranger* in his home, even if the *stranger* was a trained professional hired to take care of his wife.

Catherine suffered terribly. The postoperative complications she developed were ones I had never dealt with outside of an Intensive Care Unit. To make matters worse, Mr. Brady didn't accept or even seem to understand the reality of what was happening right before his eyes.

One morning I arrived for my scheduled visit to find him pacing in the driveway, cursing loudly at me. He assumed wrongly, as he did every day despite my frequently repeated instructions to the contrary, that I would be there all day. Here it was eleven a.m. and he was late for his golf game. He drove off in a huff and left me alone with his wife.

I ran to the sunroom and found Catherine sobbing. She begged me to send her to the hospital. She said she no longer believed hospice was right for her. She was left all alone in her house most of the time. She cried on my shoulder, saying she couldn't die because her pain was so severe, yet she was terrified to use her pain medication because it made her too sleepy to care for herself. Catherine told me the Hospice Nurse Liaison promised her she would die within a few days and that was the only reason she agreed to come home—the *only* reason, she repeated. It had been over two weeks and there was no end in sight. My heart broke for her.

As Catherine requested, I dialed her doctor's number and held the phone to her ear.

He listened to Catherine's story and then very sympathetically replied, "Yes, absolutely. I'll arrange to readmit you to the hospital this afternoon."

I watched relief flood Catherine's face. She took both of my hands in hers and brought them to her lips in gratitude.

I made what I thought would be a routine call to my supervisor, merely to inform her of Catherine's wishes and tell her about the physician's order to admit Catherine to the hospital. My supervisor flatly and inexplicably, refused to allow me to transfer Catherine to the hospital. I was stunned. Why on earth would my supervisor want Catherine to continue to suffer? As we argued quietly over the phone, I attempted to shield Catherine from the bulk of the conversation.

My supervisor sent one of the hospice social workers to meet me at the house to assess the situation and discuss the matter. He politely asked Catherine how she was feeling. Very distressed, she told him the same thing she told me, she wanted to die in the hospital. She no longer wanted hospice services. The social worker pulled me aside and informed me that our hospice supervisor would not agree to the transfer.

My reply was, "It's not up to her. It's up to Catherine."

Beside myself with concern for Catherine's well-being, I headed out to my car. Leaving Catherine alone, I sped to the office to confront my supervisor. The social worker followed me. Unfortunately for Catherine, this wasn't the first time my supervisor and I had butted heads.

OVER THE YEARS, hospice, of necessity, has become a business. Like every other segment of the healthcare industry in the United States, every hospice is regulated and reimbursed by Medicare, state agencies and private insurance companies. In addition, each hospice must follow federal, state and local guidelines, laws and licensing rules and regulations. Every hospice has employees, benefited and otherwise, who must be paid and almost every hospice works with limited resources that must be allocated. Unfortunately, many hospices operate at a loss and depend upon donations and fundraising to meet their yearly operating budget.

My supervisor and I never discussed the business of managing a hospice. That was not my concern, although in this particular instance, now I can see where concerns about funding or possible donations could have contributed to my supervisor's refusal to allow Catherine to return to the hospital. Our problem back then as I saw it, was my independent streak and her perceived need to rein me in. I disagreed with my supervisor on more than one occasion. However, up until Catherine's case, I had always deferred to her, out of respect for her extensive experience as a hospice nurse and simply because she was my boss.

THE MOMENT I became a hospice nurse, I took to heart the hospice philosophy regarding "End of Life Care." It is patient directed, or if the patient is incompetent, family directed. Occasionally, the best interests of the patient may even conflict with the interests of the family and I attempt at all times to put the needs of my patients first. I strive to keep my personal opinions to myself unless it becomes necessary to intervene in a situation I consider unsafe for either the patient or the family, or unless I'm asked. The truth is patients and their families don't always do things the way I would do them. I can accept that, but I've also come to realize not every patient, every family, or every situation is ideal, or even appropriate for hospice. It's as simple as that. Sometimes hospice staff can work with the issues involved, sometimes we work around issues, and on rare occasions, we find we can't work with them at all.

For example, on a number of occasions I have admitted patients who insist upon taking a shoebox full of unlabeled or expired medications every day. At times these are medications that are doing them no good and may be making them sick. But the person is comforted by his or her routine. While I might make suggestions and do some patient education, ultimately, I must leave the decision up to a competent patient.

At the opposite end of the spectrum, I have patients who refuse to take any medication including pain medication, preferring to be in pain or short of breath but awake, rather than feel lethargic or even a little drowsy. Again, I leave this decision up to them. Jeanine was a case in point. She hated taking medication unless it was absolutely necessary.

I am occasionally asked by physicians to admit patients to hospice and I realize after an assessment that they are inappropriate, usually for one of two reasons. Either the family simply needs help managing the care of an elderly, but very-much-alive relative, in which case I refer them to the appropriate social service agency or back to their doctor's office, or the admission is inappropriate because the patient's issues are too complex and he or she requires twenty-four hour care, seven days a week, the type of care that can only be provided by trained healthcare professionals. In some cases, the family is either unwilling or unable to provide that kind of care at home. Catherine's situation was a sad example of both reasons.

I clearly remember one very challenging case. A young man with advanced HIV/AIDS and significant associated medical problems was discharged from the hospital to his sister's home. He required twenty-four hour nursing care, which the family could not afford. By the time I arrived for the hospice evaluation, his well-intentioned sister was bordering on a psychotic break. She'd been awake for more than five days straight.

Between the young man's tracheotomy care and suctioning, his surgically implanted feeding tube and round the clock tube feedings, his intravenous infusions and flushes, his colostomy, urostomy and wound care for his many serious wounds, not to mention routine medications, laundry, linen changes, bathing and oral care for his thrush, her brother needed something done approximately every five minutes or less. In other words, like Catherine, this poor young man had so many things wrong with him that the family and hospice couldn't manage his symptoms at home. Or rather, maybe we could have attempted to manage his care, but we would not have succeeded. In this young man's case, the family didn't have the financial resources to hire a twenty-four hour caregiver, so I referred him back to his physician who readmitted him to the hospital.

The first lesson learned in midwifery is that the most important thing about attending a birth is a good outcome, in other words, a healthy mother and baby. In the case of hospice our goals are a little different, but patient safety and appropriate symptom management are still primary. We want a good outcome, a peaceful death.

AFTER ARRIVING BACK at the office, the social worker and I sat down with my supervisor and I attempted to discuss the matter. To my shock and surprise, my supervisor was furious with me for agreeing to transfer Catherine back to the hospital.

She shouted at me, "We don't do that!"

I shot back, "Yes we do. We do it all the time when we can't manage symptoms at home. Besides, the patient is alone and suffering and she's begging to go to the hospital. She's competent. She can make this decision."

I looked to the social worker for support. I had clearly heard Catherine tell him exactly the same thing she'd told me. He stared at the floor and said nothing. My heart sank. I knew I'd already lost the argument, but for Catherine's sake I persisted anyway.

"It says in our hospice guidelines that we can transfer patients back to the hospital for symptom management. The guidelines also state that the patient can revoke hospice at any time and return to the hospital under her own volition. Catherine has the right to revoke."

I practically jumped out of my skin when my supervisor pounded both fists on the desk and thundered at me,

"Mrs. Brady will not be revoking hospice! Our patients don't revoke hospice!"

"Catherine and I both spoke with her doctor," I said desperately. "He's arranging for her admission right now."

"Call him back," she insisted. "Tell him she's changed her mind."

"No, I won't do that," I replied, knowing full well I was digging my own grave.

"This is not your decision to make," she said menacingly. "It's mine."

My supervisor was obviously seething but it seemed to me that her anger had nothing to do with Catherine, so I tried a different tack.

"This isn't about me," I answered as calmly as I could, "and it's not about whether you like me. The decision is not mine and it's not yours. It's Catherine's decision. This is between Catherine and her doctor."

"If you send her to the hospital," my supervisor replied, rage evident in her eyes and her voice, "don't come back here!"

I slumped down in my chair, stunned, as I realized what she was threatening. I was still willing to go to the mat for Catherine, transfer her to the hospital and lose my job but at that moment my supervisor reached for the phone. I knew she was calling the doctor, pulling the proverbial *mat* right out from under me.

I heard her tell him, in a voice dripping with honey, that she was so sorry to bother him, but the nurse had overreacted, the situation was under control. Catherine would be staying home. She laughed apologetically as they shared a little joke at my expense.

She turned to me. "You will go back there and you will convince Catherine that we can take care of her at home." She shoved her finger in the social worker's face. "And you go with her to make sure she does it."

This was and always will be the very worst moment of my professional life.

I'd never before had a problem of any kind with a supervisor. I'm bright and I'm a quick study. I'd always worked hard and I'd been an effective, efficient, reliable, honest and compassionate nurse. I don't whine and I don't call in sick.

Never in my entire nursing career had a single person complained about either my professionalism or the quality of the care I provided. There was no question in my mind that this woman felt I was too emotionally invested in my patients and I knew I was way too independent for her taste, but her opinion of me had no bearing on Catherine's situation. As far as I could tell, she seemed unable to separate the two. Perhaps my supervisor thought of me as a loose cannon, while I saw her as a poisonous black widow spider sitting on her web, pulling all the strings.

Since that afternoon in her office, I've worked as a temporary director for another hospice. I'm willing to concede that there may have been a reason for my supervisor's reluctance to return Catherine to the hospital, most likely a financial reason. Whatever her reasoning, my supervisor could have shared her concerns with me. I was Catherine's case manager, after all, and when it came to keeping Catherine safe and pain-free, the buck stopped with me. Unfortunately my supervisor offered no justification for her decision. She shrugged aside Catherine's own desperate request to return to the hospital and she chose to ignore the extenuating circumstances regarding her lack of care and supervision at home.

As I sat in my supervisor's office that afternoon, listening to the venom spill out of her mouth, all kinds of thoughts raced through my head. Did I dare call the doctor again and try to convince him of the truth? He didn't know me from Adam, but my supervisor had maintained a very cordial working relationship with him for years. Not only did I risk making a nuisance of myself, my only recourse would be to accuse my supervisor of lying. I assumed that wouldn't get me very far.

Did I call our Hospice Medical Director and ask him to intervene? What would I say to him? Would he take my word over that of my supervisor, especially if the social worker refused to back me up? Why should he? I considered calling a state regulatory agency to report this abuse, but that would destroy Catherine's privacy in her final days, potentially undermine the reputation of an excellent hospice, and I would be forever labeled a whistle-blower. It didn't seem like a viable option.

Should I insist my supervisor accompany me to Catherine's house so she could hear what Catherine had to say firsthand? I asked if she would make a visit to Catherine. That was a dead end, she refused to accompany me. Did I resign on the spot and leave Catherine to her fate? Did I send Catherine to the hospital despite my supervisor's orders? Lose my job for insubordination and run the risk that the emergency room would send her right back home when they contacted my supervisor and Catherine's doctor for confirmation regarding the admission?

I felt stuck between a rock and a hard place, in a no-win situation. I didn't do any of the above. What I did was return to Catherine's bedside, accompanied by the social worker, put on my best face, and assure her it would be all right, we would take care of her at home. I watched the light of hope drain from her face.

Catherine whispered, "Okay," and she turned to the wall.

I felt sick. I was the biggest coward, the biggest heel, on the face of the earth. As Catherine withdrew from me, I pressed my hand to my chest, feeling the lie I'd just told squeeze like a fist around my heart. I honestly didn't know how to make things better.

Over the following weeks, I couldn't sleep. I couldn't eat. I found myself obsessing about Catherine's situation constantly and spending most of my time with her, which significantly impacted my other patients. The only bright spot was that after a week of wrangling, the social worker and I finally convinced Catherine's husband to hire a *sitter* so a responsible adult would *sit* in the home while he was off doing whatever it was he did. Catherine lasted another couple weeks. In the time remaining she hardly spoke to me.

Catherine's case destroyed any remaining shreds of a relationship I had with my supervisor and we could barely be in the same room together. The matter came to a head one morning when she shoved me out of a chair during a staff meeting after she'd just engaged in a blistering argument with our medical director. I had no involvement in the argument whatsoever, I simply happened to be the closest target and I bore the brunt of her wrath. Despite the shock I saw register on everyone's face, no one in the room spoke up on my behalf. As a matter of fact, my co-workers looked away as quickly as possible.

Terribly upset and at my wit's end, I sought out the director of human resources and spoke with her about the situation. I didn't mince words. After listening to what I had to say, she dismissed me with the helpful suggestion that I *pray about it*, because that's what she did when she had a problem.

Several days before Catherine died, I turned in my resignation. Despite the harassment I suffered, foremost in my mind was the fact that I couldn't work for someone who disliked me so much she would treat a helpless, dying patient callously simply to make a point. At least that's how her behavior seemed to me. I prefer to think her reasons had to do with me, rather than believe she disregarded

Catherine's wishes because she wanted the donations that would pour in after her death. I kept in touch with the nurse who took over the case, and she told me Catherine died a very bad death.

I left the job traumatized and depressed. For months afterwards, I tossed and turned in bed at night, replaying everything that had happened with Catherine. I despaired over my role. We at hospice were supposed to support Catherine, to be her advocates. I was supposed to be her advocate. Instead, Catherine's own wishes and needs were sacrificed and where she died became part of my supervisor's personal agenda. I felt as if I allowed it to happen. I betrayed my patient's trust. How dare I call myself a hospice nurse? Hospice is all about respecting the patient's decisions whenever possible, but Catherine's death was arbitrarily and unfairly taken out of her hands.

All I can say now is, I'm sorry. I have never let anything like that happen to another patient.

Six weeks after Catherine's death, I received a call from a hospice in a neighboring county. I'd once transferred a patient into their area and I had made a friendly connection with a couple of the nurses. I'd even completed an application the previous year, but I'd never heard from them and I had forgotten all about it. Though the manager made me an excellent offer, the thought of stepping into the home of a dying patient literally made me sick to my stomach. The experience with Catherine was so devastating I considered leaving the nursing profession altogether.

It took me several weeks of soul-searching, but I finally admitted how much I missed the work. I decided to give hospice one more try; to give myself one more chance to get it right. I accepted the job. It was a good decision. It's how I met Angel. She healed me and she taught me how to fly.

3: Second Chances

Sometimes the Bear Eats You

MALIGNANT GLIOBLASTOMA MULTIFORME, is a primary adult tumor of the cerebral hemispheres, known around our office as a *glio*, for short. The symptoms we see are usually due to increased intracranial pressure from the tumor mass, and/or associated cerebral edema and destruction or compression of brain tissue. Basically, a glioblastoma takes up the limited space available in the skull, causing swelling and tissue death. When there's too much tissue death, critical systems shut down and the patient dies, or when there is no longer room for the brain, the patient dies.

I hate glios. They inevitably happen to the nicest people, college students, young mothers, scientists and saints. Always. I can't explain it, but a glio doesn't seem to choose its victims at random. It stalks very specific people, exceptional people with tremendous potential. We all have a lot to lose but glios seem to have particularly discriminating tastes in that they prefer to kill the people who might, say, find a cure for breast cancer, or win the Nobel Peace Prize, or discover a way to reverse global warming, or develop an AIDS vaccine, or become the best baseball player to ever live, or Mother of the Year, or be elected Pope.

My hatred of brain tumors knows no bounds. The disease has no respect. At least lung cancer just kills you, a glioblastoma steals your mind first, and then it kills you. A glio is an alien parasite in an otherwise healthy body. The devastation wrought by a glio on the victim and the family is hard to imagine. Picture it as a tumor-tornado, destroying everything in its path. Worse yet, like airplane crashes, glio patients seem to come in clusters. Tumor-serial killers. Damn, I hate glios.

The saddest cases, of course, are kids. Inevitably, these kids are good students, athletic, outgoing and friendly, well-liked, just plain, ordinary nice kids. Their health histories are typically unremarkable. They are often unusually healthy children.

I once made the initial hospice contact with three young people in three days.

Monday, I saw a fourteen-year-old middle-school student. Tuesday was a straight-A university student. Wednesday was a young Dominican priest.

You walk into these homes and the kid is sitting in a wheelchair, hands shaking, head drooping, saliva dripping slowly out the side of their mouth because half their facial muscles are paralyzed or their swallow muscles are weak. The parent or brother or sister or girlfriend or boyfriend is holding their hand and wiping their face with such love and heartbreak in their eyes that it's all you can do to remain upright. You want to dissolve into a puddle on the floor and never get up again. You search desperately for a cave deep inside your mind where you can hide, because of the pain and the overwhelming sense of impending loss and the great, cosmic injustice of it all.

I walk into these rooms and my heart is ripped from my chest with just one glance. In silence, I rant and rave at God and beg Him for magical powers to stop time and reverse the disease process and prevent the inevitable death. I honestly don't know how families survive this. I doubt I could.

For instance, how do you survive the death of a woman like Angel? She was young. She was beautiful. She was an athlete. She'd built a successful business and had a promising career ahead of her. With a devoted, loving husband, two amazing children, doting parents, aunts, uncles, brothers, sisters, cousins, friends, a beautiful home, she had it all. And to top it off, she got herself a glio. See what I mean?

Angel was probably my most emotionally challenging case. Retrieve the *Terms of Endearment* out of your video file and fast forward to the scene where the Debra Winger character has to tell her children goodbye from her hospital bed and the youngest boy just shatters. Then play it over and over again. Every single visit was exactly like that, only worse, because it was real.

Angel was the bravest person I have ever met. She personified the word courage. Death was coming. She knew it and she never once looked back, or felt sorry for herself. She didn't blame anyone. She didn't even blame God. In the brief time she had left, Angel video-taped messages for each of her sons, helped her husband establish college accounts for their children and arranged for meals to be delivered by friends and family for months after her death.

Angel went ahead and reserved space for next summer's family camping trip because she felt her husband would be too distraught to do so after her death and she had vowed to keep things as normal as possible for the kids. She recruited friends to be sideline cheerleaders at her sons' soccer and basketball games, the games she would never see.

This was one of my first cases with the new hospice

and I literally broke down the moment I met Angel. She initially had another RN case manager who went off on vacation, leaving her in my capable hands. Uh-huh. Right. She should have warned me. Utterly unprepared, I walked into the bedroom. Angel sat propped up in bed, knit cap on her bald head, prednisone moon-face smiling at me, welcoming me into her room, one single room that seemed way bigger, a room that seemed as if it encompassed the whole world.

Angel's husband, Todd, was busy organizing medications and supplies at the foot of the bed. Her sister and several friends sat on her right and her left, helping her apply make-up and massaging her hands. Her father sat near her feet, painting her toenails pink, his head turned away from the chattering women, tears streaming silently down his stricken face. A video of a recent cruise trip played on the television. I watched a beautiful Angel with a full head of long, red hair, leaning against the railing of the ship, waving and smiling at the camera, while the boys clowned in the background. Angel's husband taped it because he knew it would be their last vacation together.

The boys ran in and out of the room, asking boy questions like, "Can I play video games with so and so?" "Can I go over to so and so's house?" "Where's the basketball?" Such normal everyday stuff in the midst of a situation that was so not normal. In the background, I could hear Angel's mother and aunt puttering around the kitchen, ostensibly making themselves useful but in fact avoiding the bedroom scene as much as possible.

Two things doomed me right there in the doorway, the tears on her father's face and the music her friends had chosen to accompany the video. They played the soundtrack from the movie with Bette Midler and Barbara Hershey, *Beaches*, a movie about two best friends, one of whom dies. The song playing when I walked in was "Wind Beneath My Wings." Coming on the heels of my experience with Catherine, that song just about did me in.

Without even a how-do-you-do, I burst into tears. The room suddenly became deathly quiet. I knew I'd crossed the invisible nurse-crying line. Angel motioned me over. When I bent down she put her arms around me, pulled me to her and whispered, "It's all right. I'm all right." That's when I totally lost it and ran out.

Yeah, what a great hospice nurse I am. Angel's father followed and caught up with me on the porch. I crumpled onto the front steps, my head in my hands, weeping uncontrollably. He sat down and leaned against me. Despite his own tears, he patted my back soothingly and whispered, "It's okay. It happens to all of us."

We were two complete strangers made instant companions by sorrow. It wasn't even my sorrow. Angel's death had nothing to do with me personally and yet everything about her situation was instantly and terribly personal. Angel wore the face of anyone. Angel could be my sister. Angel could be my best friend. Angel could be me.

As the weeks went by, I grew more comfortable with the situation and I managed to spend a considerable amount of time in the bedroom. I could laugh and joke with Angel and her husband and their friends. I helped ease her symptoms and keep her clean and comfortable. But it never got any easier and some days were very hard.

I took a lot of cry breaks, usually accompanied by Angel's father who was understandably distraught over the impending loss of his youngest daughter. He and I spent time sitting together on the front porch. I wish I could say I consoled him, but the truth is consolation was more of a mutual affair. We both despaired over Angel's death and the impact it would have on all the people who loved her and needed her. At times we were philosophical about it and we could talk somewhat dispassionately about what was to come, discussing the existence of heaven and comparing various philosophies of life and death. Mostly, we just hung out together because that's about all we could do in the face of what we both clearly knew would be a tragic ending.

Angel's father once said to me, "You get married and you have kids and all your love and your hopes and your dreams are centered around those kids. You want the best for them, nothing less. And if you're very, very lucky and you've done your job, you get such joy out of watching them grow and succeed and raise their own kids. Angel is the very best daughter a father could have. I never thought something like this would happen. It never even occurred to me. A parent shouldn't have to think about this. A parent should never outlive his child."

I remembered hearing my own grandmother say exactly the same thing when both my uncles were ill at the same time. My mom was a tail-ender, so her two brothers were much older than she was. I think her oldest brother was twenty when she was born and her other brother, eighteen. My grandmother lived to be eighty-six and both her sons managed to survive her by barely a year. I guess even when you're eighty-six, you feel the same. A parent should not outlive a child. But sometimes life is lived out of order. Sometimes life is so sad. Strange as it seems, it's the times when things can't get any sadder that your heart feels so very full of love it could burst. That's how it felt with Angel.

Angel was such an open person and death had so shined and polished her that now, at the end of her life, no one was excluded from her glowing circle. She'd built her circle out of love. Even the Fedex guy who delivered the hospice medications was included. It was a terrible and a poignant thing, to lose Angel and at the same time, feel her own loss. She would never see her boys grow to adulthood or watch them graduate from high school and college. She wouldn't walk down the aisle at their weddings or hold her grandchildren. She'd never bake another batch of cookies, cook a turkey on Thanksgiving, wake up to the joy of Christmas morning. Whenever I walked into the bedroom I could feel my heart turn to ice, yet Angel melted it. One look at her, one hello and I was beyond railing at her fate, at her cancer, at God. She was touched by grace and through her, so was everyone involved in her life.

The end came too soon, but Angel wore an upbeat face for her boys. They needed their mom to pretend she was just ill, not dying. Her sisters and her friends helped her with this task, searching stores all over town for brightly colored beanies and baseball caps. They made sure to pencil in eyebrows every morning and put some pink on her pale lips and cheekbones before the boys woke up.

Angel refused a hospital bed because it wouldn't hold the people she loved and she wanted everyone dear to her as close as possible in those last days. On a good day, we could pile over a dozen laughing people on her queen-sized bed. Everyone would squeeze together to get a piece of her, as if a mere touch of her gown would transfer some of her courage to us, heal us of all our ills. It was like attending a home birth where everyone crowds around the birthing mother to share in the joy of bringing a new life into the world. Only Angel was being born into the next world.

Let's face it, we all want a little slice of heaven and the door opens twice for most of us, birth and death, and then we get just a glimpse. As a hospice nurse, I get to experience it more often than most people. That doesn't make it any less holy or any less hard.

Like the majority of young, otherwise healthy people, Angel lingered. It's very difficult to let go when you are leaving so much behind, especially children. She kept her boys glued to her side until she didn't know them anymore.

Even then, they continued to kiss her hands and stroke her pale face. Watching their loving gestures broke my heart into infinitesimally small pieces. Before I met Angel, I couldn't have survived such a wrenching scene. *Old Yeller* and *Bambi* just about do me in and they are on my long list of movies to *never see again*. To this day I can't get through the spider's death scene in *Charlotte's Web*, but I toughed out Angel's death.

On the final day, after what seemed like ages, surrounded by all the people she loved, Angel took her last breath. We let out a collective sigh. We'd been holding our breaths, waiting for her to let go. No one cried. No one spoke. For a long while, no one moved. Her presence remained very strong and we were all reluctant to disturb that. Someone, somewhere, must have made a phone call, because neighbors began trickling in and Angel's home quickly filled up with friends. A priest appeared. I was familiar with Father Daniel, he'd attended a number of deaths with me, and I felt relief when Todd handed the boys and his father-in-law into Father Daniel's care so that Angel's sisters and the Home Health Aid and I could prepare her body for the mortuary.

Eventually, we sent the boys off to a friend's house and away from the permanence of their mother's death. While we waited for the mortuary van, Todd and I ended up in the driveway. We shot some hoops for a while in silence; then we played a game of Horse. His brother joined us and I backed off and let them play a much rougher game of one-on-one. They needed to play. For a few moments they needed to do something normal, something that didn't involve illness and death. Then Todd, who had been a rock for weeks, suddenly hurled the basketball down the street and lost control there in the driveway. There was nothing any of us could do but hold onto him. His brother and I held onto him for dear life.

A WEEK LATER I was still recovering from Angel's death when my own life intervened. My youngest daughter and I headed off on college trips. Several of the schools we planned to visit were in out of the way places. We were scheduled to fly on some pretty small planes into weather that was already fourteen below without even taking into consideration the wind chill factor.

B.A., before Angel, I was afraid to fly. I do not like small, enclosed spaces. I'd become accustomed to drugging myself into oblivion in order to get on a plane. But as we prepared to board our flight in Sacramento and I felt the usual panic start to build, I heard a voice say very clearly, "If I can die, you can get your ass on that plane."

Whuuuuh?

I recognized the voice immediately and turned every which way to see her, but she wasn't there. Apparently, she'd become my own private Angel. Laughing out loud, I boarded the plane.

My daughter and I flew all over the Midwest and Upper Midwest for three days in beaten-up airplanes with broken seats and tray tables that hung by a single screw, and I never gave it a second thought. We had the best time. Six months later, when I flew by myself to a wedding in Toronto, I knew I was cured. Angel did that for me. That's the kind of person she was, thinking of others even from the grave.

Angel was a teacher of the highest order. What did she teach? That life goes on when you wish it would stop. That the sun rises the day after your wife and your mom and your daughter dies. Survivor guilt is counter-productive. Her husband lived, she died. Her parents lived, she died. Both Angel's husband and father would have traded places with her in a heartbeat. That option was obviously unavailable but even so, Angel made it very clear to both of them that she accepted things the way they were and in fact, wouldn't have it any other way. Angel was no martyr. She was a realist. Some things in this world can't be fixed. A treatment-resistant glioblastoma is one of them.

Angel gently guided her boys toward a future without her, working closely with their teachers, coaches and enlisting relatives and friends to be her surrogate mothers. She planned ahead, long before she became bed bound, while she still seemed healthy. Her confidence in the boys allowed them to feel confident in themselves. She used her own inner strength to instill in them a sense of independence and competence. What a terrible thing to be forced to do, push away the people you love the most. Angel wanted her children to remember her but more than that, she hoped they would thrive even after she was gone.

Angel taught all of us involved with her that love is the most alive thing there is this side of the grave. She taught me that I didn't hurt Catherine on purpose. Sometimes when we mess up there's no time left to say we're sorry and we have to live with that. She gave me the opportunity to forgive myself, a second chance to do better. She taught me to fly.

THERE WERE OTHER glio patients I loved as well, like Father John, the gentle, selfless Dominican priest who continued to welcome me into his room at the Rectory by wiggling his toes when he could no longer speak, or even open his eyes. Christopher the twenty-year-old dear, sweet, college chemistry major, who was so worried about his mother that he visited me in my home after his death, which happens sometimes, and he asked me to tell her he was okay, more than okay actually, he looked great.

There was the young basketball phenomenon, Gina, who somehow eluded death but not before the glio stole her brain anyway and left her body withering, even after five years, in a nursing home. And there was Erica, whose new husband was so overcome by his loss that he had to be hospitalized on suicide watch.

Call it anthropomorphism on my part, but I think there is a very special place in hell reserved for glios.

4: Stories from the Trenches

Mrs. Fitzgerald

OH, THE PLACES I'VE BEEN.

Mrs. Fitzgerald lived and died in a meth lab. Her two sons managed her meds, in a manner of speaking, and two strung out prostitutes who lived and worked in the back of the house, managed her care. In other words, her sons, when they were available and could find the medication, gave her morphine for her pain and shortness of breath, while Lorena and Mary made her meals, fed her and changed her Attends when they weren't working in the back or throwing up in the bathroom because they didn't have the money to score heroin. Their hearts were in the right place.

My first visit was less than stellar. For one thing, I made the innocent mistake of parking on the court in front of Mrs. Fitzgerald's house. As soon as I got out of my car, carrying my nursing bag, a somewhat unkempt gentleman came running toward me. I learned he was one of Mrs. Fitzgerald's sons, Albert, and he yelled at me to park around the corner and walk up. I guess the neighbors didn't want anyone who went into Mrs. Fitzgerald's house parking on the court. Albert said I might find myself in some trouble.

Uh-huh. Not a good start.

By the time I came back around the corner on foot, Albert had vanished. As I skirted the garage and headed toward the front of the house, out stepped the biggest, ugliest man I'd ever seen. His clothes were black leather. Around his waist was a black leather nail-studded belt complete with two large hunting knives. Another lethal-looking knife was slung on a strap across his chest and there was a bulge under his leather vest.

We eyed each other suspiciously, then he looked me up and down, leering in a very lecherous fashion, and he smiled. Maybe he didn't actually smile. Now that I think about it, the movement his mouth made could not by any stretch of the imagination be mistaken for a smile. My stomach clenched. My vision narrowed and I prepared to either run or fight for my life.

It's funny the things you think about at times like these. All I managed to focus on was his mouth and no matter how I tried, I couldn't shake an image of being raped by a *toothless* man. I was unable to tear my eyes away from his gums. Not a particularly funny scenario I know, but as I stood there, I felt a hysterical giggle building inside of me. As if on cue, Albert came running from the house, shot the man a look of warning, grabbed my arm and dragged me inside.

As I entered the house, I sucked in a big breath. Big no-no! I quickly learned there are toxic chemicals used in the making of methamphetamine. Eventually I stopped coughing and peered through the darkness. The living room was lit by a single, low-wattage bulb that hung from a cord attached to the ceiling. Every window had been covered over with cardboard or wood and the sliding glass door in the back, which took up an entire wall, was painted black. Just then, the aforementioned sliding door slid open and a naked man stepped out. He stood there staring at me.

In a manner that I found rather dignified considering the circumstances, he exclaimed, "Oops!" and disappeared behind the door. And then it occurred to me, *who the hell admitted this patient to hospice?* I was about to storm out when I noticed the pile of ragged blankets on the couch. *Oh my God, could there possibly be a human being buried beneath them?*

I freely admit that I was terrified to cross that room. For all I knew, Mrs. Fitzgerald was dead under those blankets. Maybe dehydrated like the mother in *Psycho*. Or I might step on a rat. But by God, it was my job to find out. So I marched across the room and using only my fingertips, gingerly pulled back the crumpled bedding and sure enough there she was, still breathing.

That did it! Out of the corner of my eye, I caught Albert sneaking away. I pointed at him and said, "Stop right there. Get over here, young man. Get over here now."

I pointed to his mother. "This is not acceptable!"

Albert cringed, and tail between his legs, made his way ashamedly toward me.

Weak as she was, Mrs. Fitzgerald pleaded with me to allow her to remain in her home. If we called Adult Protective Services or if she was removed, the boys would be evicted at best, but more likely arrested. Once she was dead, she would no longer be able to protect them but she was determined to give them time to find themselves another place to live. All she asked from me was to make that possible, to keep her going for one month.

Oh the dreaded ethical dilemma. I had to ask myself some tough questions about this one. My first responsibility was to my patient. Mrs. Fitzgerald, while not of sound body, was most definitely of sound mind. She'd signed her own hospice consents. She was perfectly competent to make her own decisions. But I was also responsible for her well-being. Nurses are mandated reporters. We are obligated to report abuse or the suspected abuse of any person in our care.

After a careful assessment, I determined that Mrs. Fitzgerald was not abused. However, her care was managed in a very hit or miss fashion. She had been provided with food and water and she had been kept clean, but her sons were unreliable caregivers and I had no intention of depending on any of the strangers running in and out of the house to bathe her, launder her sheets or change her diapers.

"So," I said to Albert. "You have a problem."

I laid down some ground rules. First of all, the gargoyle out front had to go, and I made it very clear that I never wanted to see him again or I would call the cops. Secondly, he needed a caregiver in the home, someone who could be counted upon to keep his mother fed, changed, clean and dry, and who would be responsible for making sure any medications were given in the correct doses to the correct person. Albert slid behind the black glass door for a moment and returned with Lorena. I learned that Lorena and her companion Mary lived and worked in the home. Of the two, Lorena was the more clear-headed. In between customers she was studying to become a CNA, a Certified Nursing Assistant.

I had a long conversation with her. "She'll do," I replied.

Over the next few days, I managed to convince Albert to crack open some windows and I bought him a few light bulbs. Equipment arrived, like a hospital bed complete with an air mattress, a bedside commode and a wheelchair. I sent a Home Health Aide out three times a week to help with bathing and laundry and Lorena helped me set up a medication system. Call me naïve but until Lorena informed me, it hadn't occurred to me to bury morphine in a big can of ground coffee. Wow, the things they forgot to tell us in nursing school!

I will say this, I don't know for sure what mind-altering substance everyone else in the house was using, but no one and I do mean no one, ever touched Mrs. Fitzgerald's pain medications. Not even when they were twitching and retching on the bathroom floor. Once and only once, when Mary was in the throes of withdrawal, did Lorena ask me if I had any extra morphine. When I told her no she never asked again and nothing disappeared from the patient's bottle. And they weren't watering it down. I checked. I call that integrity.

Mrs. Fitzgerald got her month. One night, she fell asleep and didn't wake up. Within twenty-four hours of her death her sons and their entire entourage simply vanished. I never even got to meet Albert's younger brother, unless he was the gargoyle I ran into on the first day.

I have to admit this wasn't a fun experience, but I learned a lot about myself. First of all, I learned that I could actually do it. By *it*, I mean work effectively in such an unusual household. Secondly, I learned how to keep my patient's trust. Third, I learned to shut up and get over myself. My job allows me access into the most private aspects of a person's life and unless the circumstances are exceptional or dire and someone, including myself, is in danger of physical or psychological harm, it's not my job to judge, it's my job to do my job. Mrs. Fitzgerald's situation was far from ideal but in her case, we all managed well enough. Unfortunately sometimes doing my job is easier said than done.

Mr. X and Mr. Y

TAKE, FOR EXAMPLE, the sad case of Mr. X. When I pulled up in front of the house, I knew immediately I was dealing with a family of limited means. The signs were unmistakable. The windows for instance, most of them were cracked and taped together with duct tape, and they were entirely covered with a thick, brown crud. There was no lawn. The house was surrounded by thigh-high dead weeds. Scattered throughout the weeds, I spotted rusting chunks of metal, their original shapes and purposes anyone's guess. A warped piece of plywood barely covered the gaping hole where a single garage door used to be.

As I cautiously approached the front door, I realized something was very wrong. I thought I might faint from the stench emanating from within the house. I started retching and I actually threw up in the weeds growing over the porch. Fortunately, no one inside could see out or I would have been terribly embarrassed. I ran to my car for water and made a phone call to my office for moral support. Just in case something happened to me, I wanted somebody to know where I was. Then fearful, but spine ramrod straight, I knocked on a door that, if the spider webs were any indication, hadn't been opened in years.

DOCTORS SEE PATIENTS in their nice, clean offices. Quite often, they have no idea how these people actually live, nor do many doctors necessarily care. I don't mean that as a criticism. Physicians are incredibly busy and it's just something they don't have time to get into unless the patient or a family member brings up a specific problem. It's nobody's fault. The vast majority of people in the United States die in hospitals. On the other hand, the majority of my time is spent in the home or occasionally in a Skilled Nursing Center or a Board and Care Home. It's not all that uncommon for me to visit patients who live in abject poverty.

Hospice nurses frequently care for the mentally ill or mentally-challenged who either isolate themselves, or are isolated due to circumstances beyond their control. Many of our low-income patients don't understand how to access the support systems available to them through their health care provider, local agencies, state agencies, or even the federal government. To receive assistance, a person must ask the right questions, meet with the right people, fill out the right forms and some of our patients are simply incapable of doing that. If there is no agent to act on their behalf, they slip through the cracks. And the cracks can be pretty big, like the crevasse running through the middle of Mr. X's front porch.

I STOOD ON the porch for a long time. Finally, the door opened. An unwashed man of indeterminate age led me inside. The yard was a Victorian garden in comparison to the interior of the house. Where to begin?

First of all, I could barely negotiate my way past the open door due to the piles of garbage strewn across the floor and the stacks of magazines and yellowed newspapers blocking my every step. As I carefully threaded a narrow path, breathing through my mouth to try to minimize the stench, I slipped on some unidentified liquid and nearly fell into a pile of what appeared to be dog poop. I managed to catch myself in the nick of time, fortunately, because I wasn't entirely sure the source of the poop was really a dog. I reached toward a wall for support and withdrew my hand at the last minute because of what I saw smeared all over it.

Hyperventilating now, I desperately attempted to focus on the stern voice of my old ballet teacher as it played, loud and clear, in my head. "There is a tight string running from the bottom of your feet and out the top of your skull, pulling you upright. Good posture, ladies, good *posture*. You will not fall. You will remain in an upright, balanced position." Her mantra repeated itself over and over as the man led me toward the kitchen, past rooms stacked to the ceiling with refuse. It was the middle of winter but flies swarmed throughout the house, and, Oh . . . My. . . God...

there was something dead in there! Quite possibly many *somethings* were dead in there. My stomach is sensitive and I have an awful aversion to the smell of dead flesh.

EVERYONE THINKS NURSES come complete with cast-iron stomachs. Nothing could be further from the truth. Even though we all wear our *nurse face* when dealing with the public, a lot of us puke the minute we get out the door. I know I do. Back when I was working in Intensive Care a patient came in with a gastrointestinal bleed. She was spewing out bright red blood, like the pea soup in the movie *The Exorcist*. I was three months pregnant with my second child and anything set me off. I held the patient's emesis basin. She'd vomit, I'd run out to the restroom and vomit. She'd vomit, I'd run out to the restroom and vomit, and so it went for my entire shift.

Some things in particular get to me, like the smell of coffee-grounds emesis—half-digested blood—tarry black stools, sputum in any form, and especially the odor of decaying and/or dead flesh. My delicate stomach is no secret and unfortunately, this weakness has made me the victim of much hospice-related teasing. On the rare occasions when I actually attend staff meetings, my co-workers like nothing better than to describe the most disgusting events in graphic detail, and laugh as I turn a shade of green and slowly slide under the table.

AFTER WHAT SEEMED like forever, my guide and I arrived at the kitchen. I squeezed around him, being careful not to brush up against anything. I stepped right onto the set of a Wes Craven movie. My knees almost buckled right then, but I pulled myself together because the very last thing I wanted to do was fall into whatever was all over the floor.

There at a kitchen table, illuminated by a single bare bulb dangling on a frayed cord strung from the ceiling, sat two people so covered in filth as to be almost unrecognizable as human beings. I saw a waxy, yellowed, skeletal man gripping a fly swatter in one hand and a dirt-encrusted fork in the other, and a woman, pulled up to the table in a corroded, rusted wheelchair, her face a mass of blackened crevices, her hair hanging in greasy, dark, gray-black strings to her waist, her legs grotesquely swollen to four or five times their normal size, serous fluid oozing from both calves.

A good deal of the stench emanated from her and she was covered from head to toe with black spots. When the skeletal man reached over with his fly swatter, swatted weakly at the spots on her face and roused a buzzing swarm, I realized she didn't have some sort of awful skin condition, she was covered with flies. I stood glued to the floor, sickened beyond words. Helpless to stop it, my mouth opened and I could feel a shriek of horror coming on. Before I could utter a sound, the yellow man looked at me, coughed deep in his chest, and let fly a big wad of brown sputum in my direction. Like a surface to air missile, it came hurtling toward me. I watched in terror, helpless as a newborn babe.

Somehow a miracle occurred and time slowed. During that brief reprieve, I noticed a mountain of dog kibble in the corner to my left. It seemed the safest bet. I dove for cover, my hands sinking into its crunchy depths, and the sputum flew past my outstretched right leg and exploded harmlessly onto a discarded box of sugar-coated breakfast cereal.

As I struggled, frantically trying to dig myself out of the dog food, I heard a door open and someone called out a name. It was the daughter who'd initially contacted us regarding the hospice referral. Her name was Lucy. I scrambled to my feet, brushed myself off, turned to her and blurted out the first thing that came to mind, "Lucy, you got some s'plainin' to do!"

I think she was stunned by my audacity, but I didn't care. Exactly how do you explain yourself when your parents' home stinks like raw sewage, your parents themselves look like they've stepped off the set of *The Texas Chainsaw Massacre* and the nurse you've requested is lying face down in a pile of dog food? Lucy's father was the patient referred to us, but I was pretty dang sure we could admit her mother, her brother and, if the smell was any indication, any number of other things currently dying in the house.

I let Lucy know how appalled I was at her parents' living conditions. The son who answered the door was supposed to be caring for them. To say he wasn't doing a very good job would be a gross understatement. Unwashed dishes were stacked, literally, to the ceiling. Counter space was nonexistent. Moldy, rotting food spilled everywhere. I didn't see any cats or dogs. I assumed they were dead or dying, their carcasses adding to the stench, but their feces were scattered across the floor. Who knew how many rats had taken up residence? And the bedroom, if you could squeeze through the packed hallway, was a nightmare.

The bedding had probably not seen a washing machine in years. The torn sheets were covered with blood, sputum and excrement, dried and fresh. And the bathroom, well, we won't even get into the bathroom.

My job was to assess this patient's physical condition and his safety and admit him to hospice, but I couldn't bring myself to touch a single door knob, let alone lay hands on his walking corpse. The bumper sticker WWJD kept running through my mind. I wished I was a saintly person so I could get on my hands and knees and scrub the filth off everyone and everything regardless of my personal feelings. But I'm neither Jesus nor Mother Teresa. What I really wanted was a fire hose. I may be a nurse, but I'm only human and I have my limits.

When the patient groped his way down the hall after me, hands on both walls for support, trailing bloody phlegm and shit in his wake, and he asked me to sit on his bed and help him change his pants because he had soiled himself, I reached them—my limits, that is.

I'd been inside dirty and cluttered homes before but nothing compared to this. For the first and only time in my career, I walked out on a patient. Lucy grabbed my arm and clung to me with a death grip, so I dragged her out the door with me. She begged me to admit her father. She promised to clean the house. I doubted there was any way to do that, short of burning it to the ground and I told her so. However, because I heard a note of genuine concern in her voice, I agreed to admit her father to hospice based upon his history of lung cancer and his current state of debility. But, a big but, until the environment was clean and safe, if anything happened our nurses would not make a home visit, we would call 9-1-1, for his safety as well as for ours.

This was a Friday. I informed Lucy she had the weekend to clean her parents and their house. If I returned on Monday to find things in the same condition, or even a somewhat similar condition, I would call Social Services. I was not in the mood to be generous. As far as I was concerned, while there might be valid reasons for such squalor, there was no excuse for it. This family, I learned later, was not entirely without means and even if they were, poor does not equal filth and vice versa.

I threw the signed paperwork and my nursing bag into the back of my car. Right there in the street, I removed my shoes and socks and stripped down to my underwear. I balled everything up and shoved it under my dog's car bed in the back of my SUV. I disinfected my hands, arms and face with anti-microbial hand rinse, left my report for after-hours and weekend staff and called in sick for the rest of the day.

I drove forty miles wearing only my bra and panties. Once I got home, everything, including my shoes and my bra and panties and my dog's car bed went into my brand new heavy-duty washer on the "decontaminate" cycle. If I'd had the money to waste, I would have just thrown it all into the garbage. I jumped into the shower and even after exfoliating my entire body twice and shampooing my hair three times, I could still smell that house. To my utter disgust, the odor lingered in my nostrils through the entire weekend.

It was with great trepidation and wearing a pair of old, disposable scrubs, that I returned to the house on Monday. My confidence in Lucy was pretty shaky. Up until now, she had apparently ignored conditions in the house and the challenge of cleaning both the environment and the people living in it in a mere two days was simply too much to contemplate.

I pulled up to the curb. The exterior of the house hadn't changed. Maybe a bad sign, maybe no sign at all. I tried to keep my mind open to all possibilities, but I found myself already holding my breath. Lucy opened the front door this time, and I was pleased beyond words to see large sheets of fly paper strung up about every three feet in the hallway. I glanced down, wary of what I might step on, but the floor had been scrubbed clean, exposing the original gray linoleum. The walls looked as if someone had taken a paint scraper and disinfectant to them. They'd been scraped almost down to the drywall. I turned toward the kitchen and noted that the dog food had been shoveled into a plastic trash bin. That was something. I actually had a view of the kitchen.

Now came the real test. I still had to squeeze past stacks of newspaper in the hallway and I remarked that these had to go as they were both a fire hazard and a fall risk. Lucy agreed to have them out by the end of the day. Although every other room off the main hallway overflowed with trash, the kitchen was empty, the counter tops clean, the dishes put away or stacked neatly in a drainer. The worst of the garbage was gone, but one look at the kitchen chairs told me I would not be sitting. To my great relief, Lucy mentioned that her brother had taken her mother to a doctor's appointment and her father was in bed. I asked to see him.

Mr. X looked pretty bad, his breathing rapid, his color ashen. I noticed that the neck of his tee shirt was splotched with bloody sputum. Unfortunately, he lay in the same filthy bedding I'd seen the week before. That meant I'd have to dig through those sheets to get to him. Slinging my nursing bag across my chest to keep it off the floor, I unzipped the side pocket, and after disinfecting my hands, pulled out a pair of gloves. That was the only way I was willing to touch him.

I did my job that day and by the time I left, Mr. X had everything he needed to keep him comfortable at home, including clean sheets on his bed. But unfortunately my efforts were all in vain. The following day, Mr. X started to die. His son panicked, threw him into their old pickup truck and drove him to the hospital. He was dead on arrival. His son insisted the emergency room staff perform cardiopulmonary resuscitation. Of course it made no difference.

I honestly didn't know what to think at the time, not about his death, that was expected, but about me. My immediate sense was that I failed Mr. X, that I should have done more. That maybe I should have cleaned the shit off him like he asked me to the day I met him. I view myself as a compassionate hospice nurse, and though I was not without compassion for Mr. X, the stomach-turning revulsion I experienced in his home overwhelmed every other emotion. His situation was more than I could deal with. I blamed myself, not for his death but for something, I guess for my unwillingness to touch him. Yet even after years of reflection, if I had to return to Mr. X's house, the only thing I'd do differently would be to high-tail it back to my car and call Adult Protective Services. I can take a good, hard, honest look at myself and admit that I still would not be able to touch him. Sometimes it's just a matter of self-preservation. It's easy to slap a bumper sticker on your car. *WWYD? What Would You Do?*

SHORTLY AFTER MR. X's death, I actually cared for a patient, Mr. Y, living in a comparable situation. His home was old and in desperate need of repair. The yard was so overgrown that tangled tree branches and thick shrubs blocked access to the front door. In fact, I couldn't even push open the front gate. It looked like the forest of thorns surrounding Sleeping Beauty's castle in the Disney cartoon. The only entrance to the home was via a hole cut through the garage door.

The family was of limited means. Mr. Y and his wife lived in self-imposed semi-isolation. They had no friends that I was aware of, or at least no friends who might be available to help. Their contemporaries were mostly dead or infirm. They hadn't sought any social services despite the fact that they were certainly entitled to them and definitely could have used them. Four of their five children lived out of town. Attempting to maintain their independence, they repeatedly rebuffed offers of assistance from the one daughter who lived nearby. But that's where the similarity between Mr. X and Mr. Y ended.

Even though I accessed the house through a circle sawn out of the wooden garage door, even though the family's possessions were meager and what they had was faded and worn and occasionally patched with duct tape, I felt instantly at home. Mr. and Mrs. Y may have been elderly and poor, but their welcome was warm.

On our first meeting, Mrs. Y pulled a chair up to their chipped, but clean kitchen table and patted the frayed plastic seat. She poured me a cup of steaming coffee from a stove-top percolator. I hadn't seen one of those since I was a kid. I accepted gratefully. As I completed my assessment of Mr. Y, I noted that the rooms I needed access to, the bedroom, bathroom, kitchen and living room were spotless. After my recent traumatic experience with Mr. X, I sighed in relief.

I looked forward to my visits with Mr. and Mrs. Y. We had the opportunity to develop a relationship before anything dramatic happened. So when I arrived one afternoon and found Mr. Y home alone, standing on shaky legs, barefoot, in a spreading puddle of liquid brown stool, instead of running away, I reacted.

Usually when I arrived at the home, I'd tap on the kitchen window and Mrs. Y would wave at me. She'd disappear from view to unlatch the door opening into the laundry room. I'd head through the garage, past the vintage, '57 Chevy and the neatly hung automotive tools, and let myself in.

On this particular day, I waited a long time but no one came to the window. A little concerned, I stepped through the hole in the garage door and was surprised to find the door to the laundry room unlocked. That was not like Mrs. Y. Mr. Y was bed bound and he was not supposed to be left home alone. It's a hospice rule. If the patient is incapacitated and can't leave the home under his or her own power in the event of a fire or some other emergency, he or she is never to be left alone. I also worried that Mrs. Y might have fallen and injured herself, which is always a concern with an elderly caregiver.

I called out once, twice and then just barely heard a

soft cry for help in response. I immediately kicked it into high gear because I'd once had a patient who fell and lay on the floor for four days, unable to crawl to the phone, before we figured out what was going on and convinced the police to break into her apartment. I skidded around the corner into a hallway connecting the kitchen to the living room. I'd moved Mr. Y and all his equipment into the living room so he wouldn't feel so isolated in the back bedroom. I hit the doorway and yelled out, "Holy shit!"

Standing on shaky legs, half-way between his bed and his bedside commode, with nothing to grab onto, Mr. Y began to slip into an enlarging pool of diarrhea. Without hesitation, I flew across the room, skidded feet first onto the floor beneath him, slipped into the diarrhea and lowered him down on top of me. After all, that is what you're taught to do in nursing school. When a patient is falling and you can't stop the fall, lower them onto the floor as slowly as possible, using your own body as a cushion so they won't get injured.

My very first day as a nursing student on a surgical unit, I was assisting a five foot tall, three hundred pound post-op patient to the bathroom when she suffered a *vaso-vagal episode*. In other words, she fainted.

As she began to go down, I lowered her to the floor exactly as I was taught, but then found myself trapped beneath her. We were stuck in a corner, her unconscious bulk crushing me. I couldn't breathe and had no way of reaching the call button. In a panic, I grabbed the only thing I could reach, a waste basket, and with all the strength my left arm could muster, flung it out the door into the hallway. It took six staff members to lift her limp body off me. I think I weighed all of one hundred and five pounds at the time.

Mr. Y, of course, wasn't quite that heavy but he was well over six feet tall and he had both legs wrapped in Unna's boots, cast-like dressings we wrap around the lower extremities in cases of congestive heart failure to help manage the skin issues related to poor circulation. The dressings greatly hindered his mobility.

As you can imagine, neither of us exactly wanted to be where we were, and like drowning victims, we floundered about for a few moments before I finally instructed him to hook his upper arms over my bent knees. I dug my heels into the floor and using the diarrhea as a lubricant, slid both of us toward the bed.

At that moment, in walked Mrs. Y along with their eldest son and grandson who were visiting from Australia. Mrs. Y shrieked, "I only went to the bank!"

Mr. Y burst into tears. I wrapped my filth-covered arms around him to comfort him. He turned to look at me, I looked at him and we both began to shake with laughter, while their son and grandson stared in disbelief and horror. The next thing I knew, a mop bucket full of warm, soapy water was flung over my head like it was Gatorade and I had just won the Super Bowl, which of course made us both laugh so much harder that neither of us had the strength to get up. I don't know how it happened but I remember standing on the cement patio in the backyard with my arms outstretched, Mr. Y seated next to me in a plastic garden chair, while Mr. Y's son hosed us off with a garden hose. I could see Mrs. Y through the window on her hands and knees scrubbing the living room floor.

While we were still outdoors and dripping wet, I cut all the soiled dressings off Mr. Y's legs, bathed him with soap and hot water, dried him very thoroughly, dressed him and replaced the Unna's boots, then returned him to his bed. Someone was kind enough to bring me a plastic garbage bag and one of Mrs. Y's old housecoats.

I stripped in the privacy of the overgrown backyard, stuffed my things in the garbage bag, hosed myself off again, and put on the housecoat. By the time I came back in, Mrs. Y had made everything spick-and-span. She could not have been more apologetic. Unsuccessfully attempting to suppress a grin, I patted her on the shoulder, told her it was okay, these things happen and then laughed all the way to my car. I was barefoot, wearing an old lady's housecoat, my hair dripping, my filthy clothes and shoes in a garbage bag and I needed a shower desperately. So of course I took the rest of the day off again and headed home.

I was surprised to realize I wasn't disgusted by my experience. It felt more like watching a really outrageous Three Stooges comedy *schtick*. As I drove home, I wondered about the world of difference between my reaction to Mr. X's situation and Mr. Y's. It occurred to me that for one thing, I'd had the opportunity to develop a relationship with Mr. and Mrs. Y and I felt quite protective of them. Secondly, I knew the circumstances were out of the ordinary. Mr. Y was normally very well-cared for. And third, the problems surrounding Mr. X were way too much for one person to handle. After watching the government's response to Hurricane Katrina, I'm not sure even FEMA would have been much help.

I had blamed myself for Mr. X, believing I failed him in what I thought was his hour of need. But when I lay on the floor, rolling in diarrhea with Mr. Y in my arms, I forgave myself. I realized I'm not the one who failed Mr. X. He had already failed years before I ever considered hospice nursing as a career. I had nothing to do with the way he chose to live his life. What a sad, sad way to die.

Unpleasant Surprises

AS MY RESPONSE to Mr. X would seem to indicate, I'm not a saint. I don't like every single patient. It's actually pretty rare because I can almost always find something to like about someone. When I do dislike a patient, I'm never quite sure if it's the patient I dislike, or the family, or the situation I'm reacting to. In the following case, I hated the patient and it wasn't his fault. By the time I met him, he was already dead.

At six-fifteen one chilly November morning, as I enjoyed a leisurely shower under our newly installed Rain-Head, my husband, half-asleep, stumbled into the bathroom with the phone in his hand. He waved it in my direction. "It's for you. It's your boss."

"She's calling me at six-fifteen in the morning?" I grumbled. "My shift doesn't start for more than two hours."

He shrugged and opened the glass door a crack to slide the phone through. I wasn't especially thrilled, but I wiped the suds from my eyes and took the receiver from his hand. My boss, Ellen, said the answering service had received a call regarding a recent admit. The woman at the answering service really couldn't understand much of what the caller said, but apparently something was going on with the patient, something that needed to be addressed immediately.

I commented that this sounded like a job for the after-hours nurse. After all, she's paid to be on-call until eight a.m. My boss hemmed and hawed and finally admitted she hadn't been able to reach her. Great.

"I'm in the shower," I said. "Even if I get the shampoo out of my hair right now, it will be another fifteen to twenty minutes before I'm dressed and out of here, and I'm a good forty minutes away, minimum, from any patient we have. Almost everyone else lives closer than I do."

"I know," she mumbled, "but everyone else didn't answer their phone."

"Fine," I said. "What's the number?" I repeated it once, then quickly hung up, flipped off the water and dialed the number.

I reached the patient's caregiver, his sister. She said her

brother was in terrible pain, he was having trouble breathing. And he was vomiting blood. Oh goody. The sister
sounded remarkably calm considering the circumstances
she described. I asked a few more questions, gave her some
instructions and told her I would call when I was on my
way so I could get directions to the house. I'd never seen
this patient before, in fact, I had never received a report on
him. After I hung up, I realized I didn't even know what he
was dying of. Oh well, I'd figure it out quickly enough.

I rinsed my hair and finished up in the shower, threw
on some scrubs, (fortunately as it turned out), tossed my
gear in the car and hit the turnoff to the freeway in record
time. As I approached my merge, I gave the woman another call for directions.

"Don't rush," she said without emotion. "He just
died."

Crap. I rushed anyway.

By the time I found the place, cars lined the street. I
had to park around the corner. I grabbed my bag, clipped
my nametag on since I didn't know anyone, and joined the
line of mourners streaming into the house. It didn't take
long for me to figure out which person was the sister. She
reclined regally in a recliner, supplicants at her feet and on
every side, handing her tissues, bringing ice water, making
tea, passing out pastries and in general, milling around
looking properly distraught. I had to wind my way through
the gathered hordes so I could speak with her.

I introduced myself and offered my condolences.

"Well," she announced to the entire room, in a voice
thick with sarcasm, "you took your sweet time! I thought
hospice was available twenty-four hours a day."

Shocked, my mouth fell open, but not a sound came
out. She dismissed me with a wave of her hand and orders
to: "Clean him up and make him presentable."

I could feel my cheeks burning, but I held my tongue

and said very politely, "I'm sorry, I don't know where your brother is."

She swished her hand at me and made a noise, like the noise you make when you indicate, *off with her head!* I so wanted to smack her.

One of the people hanging around led me down the hall to a closed door. She pointed and then without a word, she turned and walked away.

I opened the door slowly. I closed it again. Shit. Shit. Shit. I don't do bodies. I definitely don't do bodies. I especially don't do bodies of people I don't know who look this bad. But I have to, it's my job. I was fuming. More than anything I wanted to tell the sister she could shove it up her ass, but I couldn't. I'm a professional and that would get me fired.

I opened the door again and stepped into the room, closing the door behind me. When this was over, I knew I was going to be very, very sick. Dead bodies come in all shapes and sizes and I've seen my fair share. This was nothing like I'd experienced before. Most of the patients I care for appear peaceful after death. This room resembled a crime scene. The body of a very large man lay sprawled across a very small bed at an odd angle, as if he died locked in a violent struggle and in terrible pain. The smell of blood and vomit, urine and feces gagged me.

From the state of things it was obvious to me that this gentleman did not die a peaceful death and I wondered why his sister hadn't called earlier. Honest to God, why the hell didn't she call us? This wasn't something that just happened at six a.m. It was apparent he'd been suffering for hours. Damn her. Damn her. All I could think was, *that bitch*, we could have helped the poor man die a good death and there wouldn't be blood and puke and shit all over for me to clean up. We take care of our people. Hospice nurses don't let this stuff happen.

Nobody helped me. Not a single person in that house lifted a finger. My request for assistance was summarily dismissed by the sister. The looks of horror I received from her guests before they averted their eyes made it very clear that I shouldn't hold my breath waiting for anyone to step forward. When I suggested we notify the mortuary because they would assist me, the sister unsheathed her claws and practically hissed at me. I called my office, but it hadn't even opened yet and the only person I managed to reach was the social worker. She was supportive and volunteered to make an appearance but cleaning up dead bodies isn't in her job description.

I didn't have a basin to put water in. I couldn't find a single towel let alone a washcloth. The room was so stuffed with furniture and equipment that I could barely squeeze my way around the bed. I had to figure out how to get this huge dead man bathed, how to change the filthy sheets, including the ones beneath him, and clean the disgusting mess off the floor, the bed, the equipment and the walls, all by myself. Talk about *dead weight*. For God's sake, I'm a nurse, not a Hazmat Team! Let's just say that by the time I finished, the room was spotless, the body bathed, hair shampooed and combed and the gentleman reposed on crisp white sheets.

I left without a word to anyone. Regardless of whether it was fair or not, I hated that dead man and I despised his sister. As a matter of fact, I hated every single person in that house. The only good thing that came out of the entire experience is that I was so angry I forgot to throw up. I learned later that the patient had just been admitted to hospice the previous morning. The sister wasn't an idiot. She had enough brains to pick up the phone at six a.m., which makes me wonder where she was before then.

WHAT'S THAT SAYING, no good deed goes unpunished?

Another co-worker went off on vacation and she left me her patients. One morning, I repeatedly tried to reach a particular patient, Mr. Wilson, as he definitely needed a visit. He had multiple pressure sores and his dressings were due to be changed. I got a busy signal for several hours. Finally, concerned for Mr. Wilson's well-being, I decided to go ahead and make an unannounced visit.

I arrived at his mobile home and at first glance, it seemed like no one was home. As I approached the side door I smelled cigarette smoke. Actually, I didn't merely smell cigarette smoke; I was nearly overcome by an incredibly powerful cloud of cigarette smoke. It seemed as if the entire house was exhaling smoke.

Holding my breath, I knocked on the door and heard a voice call out, "Help! I fell and I can't get up." Under other circumstances I might have laughed. Not this time.

I burst through the door and immediately encountered thick blue smoke, a semi-solid wall of cigarette haze. My eyes watered and a wave of nausea hit, but I swallowed hard, determined to find my patient. I pressed on through the kitchen, calling for him.

Mr. Wilson lay on the living room floor, wearing nothing but a pair of very soiled tighty-whities. Bright red blood dripped from several gashes on his forehead. His hands and arms were scraped and smeared with blood, his legs cut and bruised from his repeated struggles to get up. Fortunately he didn't appear to have broken any bones.

Mr. Wilson had managed to tip over a table and grab a box of tissues so there were bloody tissues scattered over the bloodstained carpet. He'd also reached a large ashtray and a case of cigarettes. Several lit cigarettes perched precariously in the ashtray in addition to the one burned nearly to the filter in his hand and the other dangling from his lips. He had oxygen flowing at two liters continuously through his nasal cannula.

"Help me up, would ya, honey?" He extended a bloody hand toward me.

I don't think so. The man had a good two hundred pounds and ten inches on me. I backed up and flipped off the oxygen concentrator, then put out all the cigarettes in the ashtray.

"Mr. Wilson, how long have you been on the floor?"

"Since early this morning, after my wife left."

"And where is your wife?"

"Work. Listen, honey, give me a hand here."

"Mr. Wilson, I can't pick you up. You're too big and there's not enough room."

"Go get my neighbor, he'll pick me up."

"I don't think so, Mr. Wilson. I'm calling the fire department to pick you up."

"Jeez! Don't call them! With all this blood around they'll take me to the ER."

"Maybe you need to go to the ER and get those cuts looked at. I think you could use a few stitches. Where's the phone?"

"I don't know. Over there somewhere." He waved the nub of a cigarette toward the foot of the bed.

I kept my voice even. "Mr. Wilson, I'm taking the cigarettes. You are a very lucky man. With that oxygen on, you could have started a fire and burned to death. Did someone talk to you about why you can't smoke when you're using oxygen?"

"Yeah? So what? I been smoking all my life."

"And that's why you're dying of emphysema and sitting on the floor in a bloody mess, Mr. Wilson," I muttered under my breath as I searched for the phone.

Talk about second-hand smoke. If lung disease is catching, then boy, I just caught it good.

Although I got the bleeding stopped, the paramedics, when they arrived, were not any happier than I was. We convinced Mr. Wilson to get stitched up and while they transported him to the Emergency Room, I called his wife at work. Not only had she left a bed bound patient alone, she'd left him knowing full well he would smoke with his oxygen on. She'd also left her dial-up modem running so no one could call in or out, hence the perpetual busy signal. I'd had to shut down her computer, much to her annoyance, in order to call the paramedics. There was no cell phone service in their area.

By the time Mrs. Wilson arrived home, in a snit I might add, I had the worst of the mess cleaned up. I explained the situation to her very clearly. Either she stayed home with her husband, or she hired someone to stay home with him, or she placed him in a nursing home, or I called Adult Protective Services. I felt I offered her an adequate variety of choices. She wasn't especially happy with me, particularly when I brought up the smoking while on oxygen issue. What? I realize her husband was dying but did she want him to burn to death? Who knows? Maybe she did.

I KNOW PEOPLE think that doesn't really happen; it's just an exaggeration that you can catch yourself on fire with oxygen. The truth is you're not even supposed to use petroleum jelly on your lips when you're on oxygen. I once had a patient set his face on fire while smoking with a nasal cannula blowing pure oxygen into his nose.

The flame from the match he used to light his cigarette flared up and fed by the pure oxygen, ignited his beard and hair and then ran down the length of the oxygen tubing into his house. Luckily, his quick thinking wife ripped the flaming tubing off the portable oxygen tank just in time. You could follow the scorch marks from the front walkway, up the porch steps, across the porch itself, through the screen door and along the carpet all the way to the back of the house.

In this case, my patient actually remembered to stop, drop and roll and put himself out in the front yard, but he suffered first and second degree burns to his face, head and hands. Both these patients smoked like chimneys. But that was the only thing they had in common. The second patient, the one who caught himself on fire, was a nice guy with a great sense of humor and a penchant for practical jokes. Mr. Wilson was nothing of the sort.

BY THE TIME I left the Wilsons' house that first day, I reeked. I smelled so bad I did not dare inflict myself on another patient. I couldn't even bear to smell myself, so I hit the nearest Factory Outlet Center and found a bathroom. I washed as much as I could, with soap from the dispenser, including my hair. Then I rinsed out my shirt. I thought about washing my pants, but they were just too heavy to dry under the little motion sensor blow dryer. It took me an hour to reduce the stink to a tolerable level. Shoppers came in to use the facilities and looked at me skeptically, concerned that I was a homeless person. One whiff and everyone kept their distance. I was afraid someone would call Security, but I lucked out.

It was now necessary to see Mr. Wilson daily to tend to his brand new wounds. I made sure to wear scrubs and schedule him for my very last visit of the day. Although things improved, as his wife agreed to take family leave and stay with him, until his death he never stopped smoking with his oxygen on. I enforced a rule that for nursing visits, at least, no smoking. If he wanted to burn down his mobile home, he could do it on his own time, not mine. After much argument and many threats, he grudgingly agreed. Honestly, I had to gird my loins just to set foot in his driveway.

I had this ritual, I'd bring a plastic garbage bag, a

change of scrubs, another pair of shoes and socks, a large spray bottle of water, peppermint scented body wash and towels. I set it all on the hood of my car so when I was finished caring for him, I could wash off and change before climbing behind the wheel. I only took in what I needed for the visit and anything that went into Mr. Wilson's house stayed in Mr. Wilson's house. It was kind of like, *whatever happens in Vegas, stays in Vegas.*

I know Mrs. Wilson thought I was really rude. I didn't care. I thought they were both nuts. Even so, I took good care of Mr. Wilson and his wounds actually improved before he died. His death was very peaceful and in his last hour, when he was too weak to help himself, I turned off his oxygen and held a cigarette to his lips. Even when you don't like someone, you can still honor a last request. It's not my death, after all.

Of Castles and Kings

IT WAS ABOUT this same time that I found myself caring for a series of famous and related-to-famous people. Who knew they even lived around here? Certainly not me. I'm a small town nobody from Iowa. When I'm off duty, I tend to keep pretty much to myself. My life revolves around my family and my pets and I rarely have time to pay attention to *Who's Who.*

One thing I do know is that famous people and their families are just like the rest of us. Sometimes they're nice, sometimes they're not. Sometimes they get along with each other, sometimes they don't. Sometimes families tell you exactly who they are related to the minute you walk in the door. Other times you could be caring for Mahatma Gandhi, but you'll never know until a co-worker shows you the obituary.

So it was on one fairy-tale bright morning in early spring, I found myself navigating unfamiliar country roads.

My car windows were open wide to let in the warm breeze and allow me to appreciate the distinct emerald green hillsides of Northern California, a green that was broken only by patches of purple lupines and orange poppies.

I wondered where on earth I was headed. Following a hand-drawn map, I turned down a single lane dirt track and drove up into the hills. For the first couple of miles, I passed nothing but empty meadows and tumble-down fence posts. I became a little concerned about my destination when I noticed the remains of a burned-out farmhouse on my left and I realized I no longer had cell phone reception. After another few miles, the road took a sharp turn to the right and led me through a thick grove of oak trees. When it unexpectedly dead-ended in an enormous paved cul-de-sac, my mouth fell open in astonishment.

Standing before me, arranged in a neat semi-circle on the edge of the cul-de-sac, sat four small Plexiglass enclosed guard houses. Behind each guard house sat an electronic gate, and behind each of the four gates was an elegant, winding brick drive. Peering up the driveways, I could make out at least three of the *biggest* homes I'd ever laid eyes on. I'm not good at estimating square footage but I'd guess that each home was well over thirty thousand square feet, each very different from the other and each one nestled sweetly on its own tree-covered hilltop.

The door to the farthest guardhouse opened. A uniformed gentleman stepped out and motioned me over. I took my foot off the brake and rolled toward him.

"Are you the Hospice Nurse?"

I nodded.

"They're expecting you," he replied. "Right up there." He pointed at the four-story, red-brick edifice behind him.

I wanted to ask, "Who expecting me?" I was afraid the words would come out sounding way too breathless. The guard returned to his box and picked up a phone. I couldn't make out what was said but the wrought iron gate swung open on silent hinges and he motioned me through. Despite the fact that I knew someone was dying, I'm only human and I drove as slowly as I dared, trying to look in every direction at once.

What I saw of the vast estate was beyond belief. I first passed a beautifully manicured nine-hole golf course stretching on both sides of the drive, complete with a petite Disneyland-style clubhouse, neatly parked electric golf carts and lighted crosswalks so golfers could cross the brick road in safety.

Off to my left beyond the golf course, in an idyllic pastoral setting, lay a secluded lake encompassing several acres. Canoes, rowboats and small sailboats had been drawn up onto the natural appearing sandy beach. In the middle of the lake rested two exquisitely landscaped islands, one smaller than the other, connected by a high, arching bridge, painted deep red, the type you would expect to find in a Japanese tea garden. Swans floated serenely beneath the bridge, trailed by their gangly youngsters, while families of ducks and geese dozed contentedly in the warm sun, occasionally leaning over to graze on the softest looking grass I'd ever seen.

To my right I could hardly miss a full-size baseball field complete with dugouts, an equipment room, bleachers for the spectators and a netted batting cage and pitching machine. Behind the baseball field was a softball field and behind that, a sand volleyball court. I had yet to reach the base of the hill where the house perched and all I could think was, "Wow, if my kids could only see this!" I had never in my wildest dreams imagined such wealth.

As I drew closer to the hill, I passed what appeared to be two clay tennis courts, a glass-enclosed swimming pool and lap pool, and a children's playground complete with carousel, giant sandbox, climbing wall and ornate fountain surrounded by a play pool and water slide. Heading up the hill, I caught a glimpse of the garage with twelve garage doors angled out from the main house. I wondered where on earth I would park my dust-coated, beach sand and dog-hair-filled SUV.

Not to worry. As I crested the hill, a parking attendant appeared out of a cabana set in the shade of a grove of oak trees and he motioned me into one of the nearby spaces marked, *Guests*. I parked. The attendant opened my car door and greeted me politely. He offered me his arm as I climbed down. I told him I needed to retrieve my paper-work and my nursing bag from the back seat. He insisted upon getting my things. As I thanked him, I let my eyes wander over the house in front of me. I felt absolutely overwhelmed.

Toting my bag, the attendant escorted me to a very private side door. I assumed he was leading me in through the servant's entrance but no, the door opened directly into the most enchanting little cottage I had ever seen. My senses were immediately assailed by the delicate fragrance and quiet pastels of fresh flowers spilling from the over-sized Asian urns standing in every corner of the room. As I began to focus in the deliberately muted light, I noticed a multitude of colorfully dressed women gathered quietly around an enormous ivory-colored silk canopied mahogany bed. The women ranged in age from exuberant pink-cheeked toddlers, willowy teenagers, lovely young adults, slender thirty-somethings, and sophisticated middle-aged women, all the way to well-preserved and astonishingly agile elderly women. Like Alice, it seemed I had fallen down a rabbit's hole.

As I stood very still, unwilling to intrude upon the se-renity and uncertain whom I might approach, I watched my attendant set my gear down on a trestle table. He trod si-lently upon the thick carpet until he reached a particularly striking middle-aged woman. With bowed head, he whispered into her ear. She turned in my direction and motioned me forward with an elegant wave of her hand. I hesitated, feeling terribly awkward compared to the delicate female butterflies fluttering before me. I sighed, and uttering a silent prayer to all the gods past, present and future that I wouldn't trip and make a spectacle of myself, I tiptoed carefully to her side. Eyes lowered, I actually considered making a curtsey.

The woman slid her arm through mine and with a gentle, manicured finger pressed beneath my chin, tilted my head up. Her gaze was inscrutable but her deep brown eyes radiated kindness and she said, "You are most welcome here. My mother is dying and we don't know what to do. Can you help us?"

Ah, familiar territory. "Of course," I replied.

And so we got down to business.

The matriarch of this very large extended family had suffered a massive stroke and though money was obviously no object, the family felt she would be most comfortable dying in her own bed. Everyone was eager to pitch in and I never lacked for skilled assistants. The family was a hospice nurse's dream. They did an exemplary job of caring for this tiny woman. No task was too menial. They performed every action tenderly and with love.

As the weeks passed, I learned a little about the lives of the people who shared this estate. Apparently the patriarch of the family, my patient's husband, had been a self-made man. A shrine dedicated to him had been set up in a corner of my patient's cottage, complete with photos and framed newspaper clippings, in addition to candles and incense. He founded a small company that ultimately evolved into an enormous multi-national corporation. He not only provided for his immediate family of eight, but his many companies employed nearly all his relatives in addition to probably the population of a small nation. They were a very close family and several generations lived in the various wings of the home. The family members were also very close with their employees, a few outside consultants and even certain government officials from around the world. There was no shortage of important visitors during the weeks I worked with the patient.

The woman who first spoke with me, the patient's eldest daughter, explained that once a year, the family flew their scattered relatives and their executives, along with their families, in from all corners of the globe for a week of what she referred to as *the Olympics*. She said the games had originally been her mother's idea, and that her mother in particular, looked forward to the event for the entire year. Everyone was scheduled to fly in the following week and the daughter wondered if she should cancel. She said she felt torn because although her mother lay dying, she knew her mother would want the family and friends to be together. She asked me point blank how long her mother had to live. Would she be there for the games?

I asked, as I usually do, "How honest do you want me to be?"

She answered, "Completely honest."

"She won't be here," I said. "She has three, maybe four days."

We were standing side by side in the cavernous kitchen, a team of busy cooks behind us, the buttery aroma of fresh baked croissants drifting our way. She studied the floor and absently rubbed the tip of her jeweled pump along the edge of the blue slate tile.

She looked up and gave me a wry smile. "The games must go on, I guess. Whether Mom's here or not, I believe she'll enjoy them. Thank you for your honesty."

My patient lived exactly four more days, long enough for the early arrivals to pay their respects. The first day of the Olympics was postponed for the funeral service which was held in the vast meadow behind the house. All the invited guests were in attendance.

The games began as planned the following day. The daughter later told me the week was a great success and she felt her mother's presence very strongly. She asked if that was normal. I reassured her that her feelings were completely normal. Very often family members feel the presence of a deceased loved one for a long time after a death. In fact, I'm surprised when it doesn't happen.

This family was unique, in the sense that everyone came together to care for this woman. There was agreement among all parties involved. Their primary concern was that the patient be allowed to die peacefully, and everyone adjusted his or her schedule and set aside any and all personal matters to make it happen.

This case was of special significance to me, as in my experience it's very unusual for such a large family to reach this kind of consensus. Actually, this is the largest family I've ever dealt with in my practice, which made it all the more remarkable. A more common role for me is that of referee between family members. Usually some family members understand the hospice philosophy and agree with it, while other family members insist that to turn to hospice means the patient is *giving up*.

As I said, rich families have many of the same interpersonal problems as poor families; it's just that if you're rich, you don't have financial concerns in addition to all the issues related to caring for a dying relative. However, no matter which designer label they were wearing, this particular family dived right in, changed diapers and gave bed baths without complaint.

MEANWHILE, ON THE other side of the valley, I was involved with another wealthy and similarly attentive family.

This family lived on the wrong side of the tracks, so to speak. The area was a mixed bag, semi-rural, with some cultivated farmland, a few scattered rundown trailers, a couple of brand new cheap housing developments plopped down in the middle of nowhere, and a rutted, dead-end dirt road that had been ignored for decades. My patient lived on the dead-end road.

I really didn't know what to expect. I only knew that the patient, a seventy-two-year-old Hispanic male, had suffered a stroke. Feeling a bit unnerved by the isolation, I parked, grabbed my gear and picked my way up the uneven, graveled walkway. The walkway itself was almost completely roofed over by ancient, massive oaks. Some of the longer branches hung nearly to the ground.

The front porch was one of those old-fashioned screened-in Midwestern jobs that you rarely see on the West Coast. Due to the dim light and the amount of dust on the screens, once I stepped onto the porch, I found it difficult to see anything. The house itself gave off the aura of a black hole, like it sucked everything in and never let anything back out. I felt an odd chill on the back of my neck when I pressed the bell but then the door opened and I felt a chill of a different sort. This time Alice didn't fall down a rabbit's hole, I fell through the looking glass into a very intriguing place.

My escort into this world was one of the most handsome and sexiest men I have ever had the good fortune to meet. Just facing him through the open door stole the breath from my lungs and turned my insides to a pool of melted butter. The fact that he sat in a wheelchair did not detract one iota from his sex appeal.

His face looked like it had been chiseled from a creamy-gold marble, his features sculpted like the perfect Adonis. High cheekbones, straight Roman nose, masculine chin and jaw complete with a perfect five o'clock shadow framing soft, sensuous lips. He flashed a wide, white smile at some inane comment I made and when the corners of his golden brown eyes crinkled in amusement I felt it to the tips of my toes. I was seriously in danger of swooning.

Dark, unruly hair fell in a thick cascade over his broad shoulders. Some of it was braided and caught in a leather thong at the nape of his neck but most of it hung free and gleamed with mahogany highlights against the black leather back of his custom-made wheelchair. Yummy! He wore leather sport gloves, the kind without fingers and I noted almost peripherally that he was only able to use the thumb and index finger on each hand, while both little fingers were contracted and stood out at odd angles as he pushed his light-weight wheels. I realized that he wasn't a paraplegic as I'd initially thought, rather, he was a quadriplegic, but his paralysis was incomplete and he still had quite a bit of movement in his upper extremities. His upper body was, in fact, powerfully built.

Beneath his tight white shirt, the outlines of his well-developed triceps, biceps, pectorals and trapezius muscles were very visible. His legs were slender but not as stunted and atrophied as I've seen with other quadriplegics. He wore close-fitting blue jeans and Reeboks. His legs were strapped into the wheelchair with black Velcro straps. Slung around his hip, like a cowboy, was a gun belt complete with holster holding a cell phone. A pager was tucked into the front pocket of his jeans.

I was so intent upon stealing surreptitious glances at my guide that I failed to notice where he was leading me until I found myself blinking in the bright sunlight of an open flagstone-paved courtyard. Water cascaded from a terracotta fountain, spilling rainbows into the perfumed air. Statues of Greek gods were tucked into hidden niches and corners. Everywhere I looked, I saw flowers. Fat, contented bumblebees bumbled, butterflies fluttered, and honeybees were so weighed down with pollen they could barely fly. This place, like my escort, was stunning and I suddenly laughed aloud.

Out of the blue, I was overcome with a sense of the richness of life. I felt blood surge through my veins. Time stopped and so did I. I stood still, eyes closed, face turned up to collect the warm golden light, oddly content to merely be standing in this very unexpected place. My wheelchair guide accepted my sudden compulsion with equanimity, as if this typically happened to visitors and he waited patiently at my side. Then I sighed, life resumed its normal configuration and we continued on our way in comfortable silence.

This is a book about dying, right? Sometimes my work is more about living. The longer I'm around dying people, the more I love the living. I was not always a people person but I am now. My favorite shirt spouts a logo that says, *Love This Life* on the front and I wear it on patient visits all the time. I see no contradiction. Despite the death I see, I do love this life. On that day, when I stepped into that garden, I remembered exactly how much.

The courtyard was a large square and it occurred to me that each side must open into entirely separate living quarters. Once I was admitted to the main house and met the rest of the family, I gained a better understanding of how things worked. My wheelchair Adonis was named Marcus. He was my ticket to a remarkable show.

First I met Marcus' mother. Statuesque would best describe her. She had to be pushing seventy but she didn't look a day over fifty. She was tall and slender. She had a lovely, smooth peaches-and-cream complexion. Aristocratic brows arched over soft hazel eyes that belied a formidable intellect and an inner core of steel. Her hands were supple, her fingers long and graceful, her grip on both my hands firm, warm and welcoming as she guided me to the outdoor kitchen and sat me on a sun-warmed bench. She pointed out a bedroom nearby, the double doors opening into the courtyard. Gauzy yellow curtains drifted gently in the breeze. In that room, her husband of nearly fifty years lay dying.

Marcus stayed close at hand as we chatted, helping with consent forms, gently filling in the blanks during those moments when his mother was overcome by emotion.

Marcus and his mother took me to meet the patient. He lay on a pile of pillows in an enormous antique Hacienda-style bed. Sitting beside him, lovingly clasping a pale, limp hand in his big strong one, was another stunningly beautiful man in a motorized wheelchair, Marcus' younger brother, Thomas. My eyes widened and I shot a look at Marcus as I wondered what on earth had happened to both of them. Marcus merely raised his dark brows in amusement. He didn't volunteer any information.

Despite the fact that Marcus' younger brother kept his hair short, the resemblance was striking, right down to the golden eyes, the strong shoulders and the long, tapered fingers. He too was solidly built and suffered very little wasting of his lower extremities. Unlike Marcus, he was obviously a paraplegic. He too wore a sparkling white shirt and faded blue jeans, but his shoes were black Nikes. Like Marcus, he kept his legs positioned in the wheelchair with Velcro straps. He also carried a cell phone and a pager in a holster slung around his hips. The *sensitive hunk* quotient in the room had definitely moved right off the scale.

The patient himself was unresponsive. Despite his slack face, he was still a handsome man, strongly built and I could see where Marcus and Thomas got their good looks. I knew that their father would live a while yet. I completed my assessment with some gentle assistance from his sons and then Marcus, his mother and I retired to the bright, airy and very modern indoor kitchen. The room had obviously been remodeled in order to accommodate wheelchairs. Everything had been made accessible for Marcus and his brother.

Just as I pulled a heavy chair up to the ornate wooden table, the front door burst open and in rushed eight tall, extremely handsome teenage boys. I would guess their ages ranged from fourteen to eighteen. Suddenly the room was filled with backpacks, youthful male voices and laughter. Cartons of milk, cans of soda and snacks of all description appeared and just as quickly disappeared into hungry boys.

Marcus was in his element. The boys gathered around and I watched, spellbound, as he listened indulgently to all their stories and discussed homework and activity schedules with them. Who were these boys? I turned to Marcus' mother only to come face to face with Thomas who had apparently wheeled up next to me while I was focused on the boys. He cuddled a darling toddler on his lap. She had the face of a little angel, her skin alabaster, cheeks pink, her head a halo of bronze ringlets.

I wondered to myself, what kind of household was this? Who were these people? Where did they come from? What did they do? And why were these two brothers in wheelchairs?

I was bursting with curiosity despite the fact that the answers were none of my business. I managed, with great difficulty, to keep my questions to myself, but my patient's wife voluntarily filled in a few of the blanks.

The family had emigrated from another country. They still owned a great deal of property in their homeland and a third son and his family and Thomas' wife lived there to manage the holdings. She mentioned that Thomas split his time between his home there and here in the States. He'd come back because of his father's illness. The little girl was his first child. The teenagers were her grandsons. One of the boys was Marcus' biological son. If Marcus had a wife, she wasn't mentioned. The other boys were his nephews. He'd adopted them. His oldest brother and sister were both dead from drug overdoses. He had another sister living out East somewhere. My patient's wife was rather vague about her. I couldn't bring myself to ask how Marcus and his brother ended up in wheelchairs and she didn't offer any explanation. I learned much later that they had both been shot. I decided I'd prefer to remain in the dark about the circumstances.

I relished every minute spent with this family. My patient lived another five weeks and never regained consciousness, but I came to love him because of the family he'd made. The house was filled with life, joy, loud laughter and boyish pranks. The only females in the home were my patient's wife and his granddaughter. Although they were surrounded by an excess of testosterone in a male-dominated world, they were cherished. The protectiveness even extended to me. It was a sort of old-fashioned way of life that I had never before been exposed to outside of the book *Jane Eyre* or in the writings of Jane Austen.

Having grown up without a whole lot of parental guidance and supervision, I'm quite independent. I learned from an early age to rely on myself. It wasn't exactly a conscious choice, but it became increasingly so as I matured. In the beginning, my self-reliance was more or less a matter of physical and emotional survival. Ultimately, it became a matter of pride, despite all the trouble I managed to get into on my own.

I had no clue what it felt like to have a man, a father, big brother, an uncle, or men, as in this particular case, look out for me. As a matter of fact, my experience with men, other than my husband, has been a mixed bag at best. I can't even claim that my husband is especially protective. He prefers me to be independent because it allows him greater freedom. If anything, having experienced some of the darker side of life, I am the more protective of the two of us when it comes to each other and our children.

It's obvious to me that we live in a society of contradictions. As women, we want our freedom and we are encouraged to make our own way, but freedom comes with a price. The simple fact is that men are bigger, stronger and have a greater capacity for violent behavior. Unfortunately, when you come right down to it, in certain situations, women are not safe.

In this patient's home, the feeling of being protected, cherished, almost cocooned in a surprisingly gentle world of old-fashioned male chivalry, was a revelation to me. Allowing myself to become immersed in their domain of shadow and sunlight gave me chills in a good way, I felt the kind of chills you feel when someone brushes fingers lightly over the back of your neck. The chills you get from listening to a soft and soothing voice when you're tired or sick, pleasant shivers. As a woman and a nurse, I felt respected in every way.

It was a revelation to be respected simply by virtue of my gender. I've been respected for my skills and accomplishments, for my intelligence, my achievements in school, for my unusual fashion sense, even for my outspokenness and occasional brash behavior, but never simply because I'm a woman. Having grown up with Women's Liberation and burned my bra years ago, a nagging voice in my brain insisted I should feel insulted. But all the other voices in my brain shouted back, "Shut up you idiot! Enjoy it while you can!"

Marcus or one of the boys inevitably came out to greet me and carry my supplies and my bag. I never struggled to complete a difficult task on my own, as has been the case with many of my patients. The bedroom was clean and organized. Fresh towels and linens were always stacked and waiting. Medications were in order and every symptom observed or medication given recorded in a journal that sat at the bedside. Everyone took his turn helping. Nobody complained. Imagine your average teenager willingly cleaning his grandfather's bottom, or learning how to change sheets beneath an incapacitated person, or giving a bed bath.

And of course there was Marcus, ever-present with that wide smile of his. He could coax laughter from a rock. His smile was ambrosia, food of the gods. I lived on it. I have to admit that Marcus did turn my head, not that I let on. Our relationship was warm, but I remained strictly professional at all times.

I remember my visits to this family and their home as if they were an hour walking barefoot in the sand of a tropical beach. I close my eyes and I can feel a warm breeze ruffling my hair, I hear the sound of the waves lapping against the shore, I can smell the briny ocean. When I remember Marcus, I haven't a care in the world. For once in my life, I didn't have to watch my back. There was always someone around to do it for me.

What a major role-reversal. It felt strange to get so much more than I gave. I'm unaccustomed to being on the receiving end, but the generous spirit of this family was so natural, so all-encompassing and so unself-conscious that it was surprisingly simple to drop my barriers and accept their world, accept them into my heart. Wow. I'm friendly with most of my patients and families, but I'm pretty guarded with my heart. Not in this case. I opened my chest without reservation and handed my heart to them on a platter.

I COULDN'T HELP but compare the two families above with the families of two patients who had died just prior to these cases. I cared for the grandmother of a famous television personality who happens to be married to an equally famous movie star, and I got caught in the middle of an awful family feud. I was actually the second nurse assigned to the case. The first nurse had been thrown out of the house for threatening to call Adult Protective Services if the patient's *difficult* elder daughter didn't shape up and provide the care the patient needed. By the time I got involved, the younger daughter had stepped in and moved my patient into her small home over the loud objections of her older sister.

The *difficult* daughter made her feelings very clear. By right of what she considered her standing on the celebrity ladder, she felt she deserved all the attention for sacrificing her valuable time to care for her mother. Except she sacrificed nothing and she took lousy care of her. She abused the hired help, the hospice staff and her poor sister, brother-in-law and their children. Lord, I wanted to smack that woman something fierce.

Ultimately and very unfortunately for me, we all came to an *arrangement*. Whenever the older daughter and her posse wanted to visit my patient, the younger daughter and her family left their home and I supervised the visit. Oh joy. What an obnoxious bunch of stuck-up . . . Once a week for three months, I had to sit through an afternoon of criticism, second guessing, and bad-mouthing by ignorant, ill-tempered, over-dressed know-it-alls, who made a point of name-dropping, shoving enormous diamonds under my nose, bragging about their famous offspring. They sneered at my baggy scrubs and ridiculed the hospice philosophy.

No opening my heart here. These people would have ripped it out of my chest and devoured it while it was still beating, given half a chance.

Despite the private jet belonging to the famous grandchild, in the three-plus months I was involved with the case this person never showed up to visit the beloved grandmother, never even called. Yet somehow, despite this person's overwhelming schedule, this person managed to find the time to fly up to our area via said private jet to pick up the rest of their immediate family for a two-week trip to the Mexican Riviera. You know how it is, we all have our priorities.

At the exact same time, forty miles away, another of my patients, the grandfather of yet another famous movie star, lay on his deathbed. Once again, the famous star couldn't find the time to pick up the damn phone. Of course in this case, we did have autographed photos sitting on the bedside table.

Really . . . I mean, come on.

When my grandmother, my mother's mother died, I was living a thousand miles away, poor as a church mouse, putting myself through nursing school. She died unexpectedly during midterm exams. My mother insisted I stay in school. I felt terribly guilty, but I consoled myself with the fact that I had been back to see her just three weeks before and we'd had a marvelous time together. I get it, sometimes there are reasons you can't come home. But as far as I'm concerned, wealth and fame do not excuse shallow, insensitive, self-centered behavior. There's rich in what counts and then there's just plain rich, and there's a world of difference between the two. I'll take rich in what counts any day. The families of my first two patients kept things in perspective and they managed to have it all. That actually gives me a lot of hope when it comes to camels fitting through the eye of a needle.

Another Mouth to Feed

"OH GOD! NOT another feeding tube!" That was my response to the report on Mr. Perez. It's my standard response. I hate feeding tubes in unconscious patients. Why? Because it's almost always the same thing, the family doesn't want to stop the tube feedings because they think the patient will starve to death and they believe his death will be their fault.

The doctor is reluctant to say anything about the tube feedings because he worries the family will accuse him of starving the patient. So what happens? The patient dies *because* of the feeding tube. Tube feedings either kill the patient outright, or the patient dies way sooner and in far greater discomfort than he or she would have otherwise. Feeding tubes quite literally give me a stomachache.

Imagine, for a moment, that you have advanced Alzheimer's Dementia. You lie in a bed all day and night. You are nothing but skin and bones. You are without any discernible self-awareness, unable to move on your own, unable to speak or hold your head upright, unable to feed yourself or swallow because your brain has forgotten how. You are incontinent of urine and stool. If you are one of the lucky ones, and you have attentive caregivers, someone will notice your smell in a reasonable amount of time and they will clean you up before your skin begins to break down and you develop a decubitus ulcer, a bedsore, that may, because of your continued incontinence, immobility and poor absorption of nutrients, open all the way to the bone.

Then someone in your family, or perhaps a member of the nursing staff where you reside, comes up with the bright idea that if you only had better nutrition, you would *feel* better and perhaps your condition would *improve*. Uh-huh. Right. *Not gonna happen.*

So, someone speaks with your doctor and asks that he arrange to insert a feeding tube.

You are taken to the hospital where you are put under general anesthesia and a tube is surgically inserted directly into your stomach so someone, with either a large syringe or a drip bag, can force cans of baby formula into you. Of course it's not really baby formula, it's a nutritional supplement more like Instant Breakfast with fiber.

I'm the first to admit that there is a time and a place for a feeding tube. When an otherwise functional person has an illness or injury that is not terminal, but it prevents him from eating or swallowing, a feeding tube may be the only way he can receive nutrition. In addition, if a person is in the midst of treatment for a condition such as a stroke or cancer and the person's ability to swallow is impaired or damaged, that's an indication for the placement of a feeding tube.

For instance my patient, John, had a feeding tube inserted when radiation treatments for his lung cancer destroyed his ability to swallow but that was well before he became terminal. He and his family made the decision early on to stop using the tube when he neared the end of his life. Most Amyotrophic Lateral Sclerosis patients have a feeding tube placed at some point, as do many people who suffer from brain injuries, tumors, or other neurological diseases. In these cases a feeding tube is essential for the patient's well-being and yes, improved nutrition in these cases can help heal a wound or an infection.

However, when a patient is dying, it is a different situation altogether. It is with great hesitation that I admit patients with certain diagnoses when they have a feeding tube, especially when the family is very attached to using the feeding tube. In my experience unless the family is willing to discontinue tube feedings, the cause of death is almost inevitably tube-feeding related drowning.

Part of the dying process is the body's decreasing ability to digest food and absorb nutrients. The gastrointestinal tract slows down and pretty much shuts off. After all, there are more important organs to consider when it comes to blood supply, the brain, the heart and the lungs. When you pour food into a stomach that is not emptying properly, if at all, where does it go? Unfortunately, it usually goes back up the esophagus and into the lungs. Debilitated patients with feeding tubes very typically succumb to aspiration pneumonia.

Studies have shown that patients on hospice who become dehydrated in their final weeks, days, or hours, die much more comfortably than patients who are kept artificially hydrated with intravenous fluids or supplemental tube feedings. As systems start to malfunction, which they always do when people die, body fluids don't stay where they're supposed to. Systems seem to become porous in a sense, so if you put intravenous fluids into a vein, the extra fluid is likely to end up in the lungs or pooled in the legs, arms, or even the face.

It's been my experience that the studies regarding hydration accurately reflect what happens with dying patients. If a patient is conscious or semi-conscious, they can ask for fluids. Even though they typically are able to manage only a small amount of liquid at one time, that seems to be enough to satisfy them. We always teach caregivers to provide oral care, to keep the patient's lips and mouth clean and moist with lubricants or small amounts of water. I tell families that if the patient loved soda or apple juice or iced tea, they can use that to refresh their mouth. Sometimes people prefer a spongy swab dipped in mouthwash or ice water.

Every single person I've cared for who did not have a feeding tube and became dehydrated has died more comfortably than every single person I've cared for with a feeding tube that remained in use until their death.

Mr. Perez's family loved him. They loved him very much. Part of loving him was that they wanted desperately to save him despite the fact that he was already comatose when the referral came in to hospice. I did my best to educate the family on the process of death and dying, but nothing I said had any impact on Mr. Perez's daughter Anna.

As Mr. Perez's condition worsened, the more liquid Anna forced through his feeding tube. Anna convinced herself that if she could just get enough nutrition into her father he would wake up and live. We fought a very determined turf battle and I lost. He may have been my patient, but I kept in mind that he was her father first.

Mr. Perez suffered terribly because of the tube feedings. During the last week of his life, his belly swelled to an enormous size because his gastrointestinal tract wasn't moving and the liquid had nowhere to go. His lungs filled with fluid, and because of that he ran very high fevers which we could not control with either Tylenol suppositories or cool baths. More than anything I wanted to rip that tube out of his belly, but I couldn't, he wasn't my father. It wasn't my decision. Undigested liquid dribbled out of his mouth constantly. Anna would pour the food in and out it would come, and then she'd pour in more.

On the morning of Mr. Perez's death, I received a call. I recognized Anna's voice, but she was screaming incoherently and I couldn't understand her. I rushed to her home, only to find her father dead, yellow liquid pouring out of his mouth and nose. He had drowned. I tried to explain to Anna that he was dead. I tried to reason with her. I tried in vain to get her to stop feeding him.

When I failed to reach Anna with words, I put a gentle hand on her arm to stop her from using the syringe to force in another can of liquid. She was pumped full of adrenalin and absolutely determined to feed her father. She shoved me to the floor. I picked myself up and raced out the door, hoping to find Anna's friend in his office. Her friend happened to be the manager of the apartment complex.

Unknown to me, upon hearing Anna's screams, neighbors had already called the police. I came around a blind corner and ran smack into a cop's chest. He grunted and took a few paces backward while I sat down hard on the cement sidewalk, the wind knocked out of me. It was fortunate that I literally ran into him. He later said that had he seen me running from the apartment, he might have drawn his gun.

I tried my best to say, "Hospice. Died. Daughter . . ." as I pointed toward the apartment and held up my name badge. I could only mouth the words.

By this time, Anna's screams had attracted a crowd. The officer helped me to my feet and he was patient enough to allow me to contact our hospice Medical Social Worker so she could intervene, and hopefully, calm Anna. The Social Worker, Teresa, arrived fifteen minutes later. Between Teresa, the police officer, two paramedics, Anna's uncle, the apartment manager and me, it took a long time to convince Anna to stop forcing food into her father's dead body and release him to the mortuary. Mr. Perez was the worst example I've seen of what can happen with a feeding tube.

I ONCE CARED for an elderly Filipino woman with esophageal cancer. She insisted upon having two cans of Instant Breakfast poured into her stomach every four hours via a naso-gastric tube, a tube inserted through her nose into her stomach. As soon as we poured the Instant Breakfast in, she became so nauseated that she insisted we hook her up to suction and suck the stuff out again. There was no reasoning with her and she put herself and everyone else through this misery for several weeks before she finally decided she'd had enough. She let me pull out the tube, and for the remainder of her life, another month, stuck with small amounts of clear liquids. Her nausea immediately vanished, she regained her innate good humor, enjoyed the time she had with her family, and she died comfortably in her own bed, surrounded by the people she loved.

Every one of us has a relationship with food, and we certainly have a deep attachment to feeding and nurturing those we love. We even feel compelled to feed complete strangers. I believe this desire to welcome people to our table is ancient, something very old within ourselves and within probably every culture in the world. It's altruism in its purest form, the sharing of food, the breaking of bread together. When we love someone, we want to feed them, especially when they are sick. How much stronger might that desire be when the person we love has a terminal condition and we're helpless to do anything about it?

I understand the impulse to feed a dying patient. Somebody is sick, they appear to be wasting away, you should feed them, that is what a good son, daughter, father, mother, husband, wife, brother, sister does. It seems counterintuitive to do otherwise. But feeding a dying person doesn't help. If there's one thing I'd like you to take from this book it would be this, feeding a dying person doesn't make them better. It makes them die faster and they suffer while they're dying. It's the kind of suffering hospice nurses can't fix because the cure isn't a gentle touch or soft words, or medications, or positioning, or suctioning, the cure is to stop the feedings.

It's like vital signs. I rarely take vital signs. In fact, I only take vital signs after my initial assessment if the act is important to the family or the patient. I know most people think it's a given, nurses take vital signs. What they don't realize is that *vital signs tell me very little when it comes to a hospice patient.* I look at my patients. By that, I mean I really look at my patients. I look, I listen, I touch, I smell, because cancer and approaching death both have peculiar odors. I reach out with all my senses and I treat my patients accordingly.

People who are terminally ill, who are approaching death, have very unstable vital signs for all kinds of reasons. Temps go up and down as does blood pressure. The important thing is how the patient appears, and if they can express themselves, how they feel. I bring up the subject of vital signs because they are a *magical* measurement people cling to, even nursing students and new grads. Nursing students and new grads are often guilty of making a decision based upon a monitor reading rather than what is actually happening with their patient. Chalk it up to inexperience, I've done it myself.

Feeding tubes often involve the same kind of "magical" thinking. Families are sometimes so busy clinging to the false hope a feeding tube offers that they can't see what's right in front of them. Your father is dead and food is coming out of his nose.

Anna's not alone. It's a tough decision to remove a feeding tube once it's been inserted, or to stop feedings, or to resist the desire to insert a feeding tube in the first place. Remember, the reason people are referred to hospice is the terminal nature of their disease process. The natural outcome of any disease process we see, with very few exceptions, is death. A feeding tube doesn't change that fact. From my point of view, it just means a shorter length of stay on hospice.

A Scary Mix

GUNS AND CANCER don't always mix. It's rare, but I have been involved with families where there are guns, distraught family members and dying people and it is not pretty. On one occasion, I found myself trapped in a bedroom with my unconscious patient while her husband ranted and raved, paced and threatened in the doorway. I was flat out terrified because the house was a damned arsenal. Knowing the patient and her husband as I did, I figured the odds were better than fifty-fifty that the situation could escalate into a murder-suicide. I didn't want to be on the murder end of things simply because I happened to be present.

My patient's husband was looking for someone to blame for his wife's illness, the doctors—the nurses, the neighbors, the government. Because I recognized a powder keg and a short fuse when I saw one, I was always respect-ful, trod lightly, and watched my mouth. Fortunately, he didn't blame me. He felt I'd always listened to his concerns. Unfortunately, he wasn't about to let me out of the bed-room while he openly considered his very drastic options.

I sat at his wife's side, carefully keeping my expression mild, caressing her hair with gentle hands, smoothing her brow, massaging her temples, doing my best to soothe him vicariously. Other than that, I stayed very still. Pretending he was a cornered animal, I remained calm and I spoke in a soft, low voice. I validated everything he said, reflected his own words back to him and did my best to exude empathy. I was convinced that the only way I was getting out of that house under my own power was to keep his attention and stay connected with him.

It took almost two hours, but he finally allowed me to leave the bedroom. Then he insisted that I accompany him into his study. For another hour, he sat with his back against the closed door as he opened up about the insanity of his early life, the stability his wife had provided, and how devastated he was by her cancer and approaching death. He finally broke down and sobbed on my shoulder. He agreed to let me call his parents.

I coaxed him out onto the front porch and sat by his side, holding tightly to his hand until they arrived. After speaking with his parents and getting their guarantee that he would never be left alone and the weapons would be removed from the house, I decided against involving the police. The man trusted me, I couldn't abuse that trust. My legs shook as I walked to my car, but I made an effort to wave and smile as I drove away. I turned the corner, pulled to the curb and collapsed against the steering wheel, shaking with my own uncontrollable sobs.

After meeting with the entire hospice staff and discussing our various options, we decided to keep the family on service, provided no one involved with the case ever felt threatened. I was never again alone with the patient and her husband. My patient died very peacefully, her husband handled it about as well as you might expect. I left the house as soon as I felt things were under control and drove away, relieved, without a second glance.

ON ANOTHER OCCASION, I made a routine visit to an elderly couple. The husband was dying of cancer. I didn't know him well even though he'd been one of my patients for several weeks. The gentleman was obviously depressed and very uncommunicative. His wife was friendly enough, but she had her own health problems and caring for her taciturn, bed bound husband was a challenge.

At my knock, she flung open the door, grabbed me with surprising strength and whispered hoarsely that her husband had a loaded gun in the bedroom. She said he'd crawled out of bed the night before, pulled it out of a locked cabinet, loaded it and every time she tried to enter the bedroom, he waved it in her direction. He said he'd shoot her and then himself if he heard her on the phone.

Despite the fact that the woman was swollen to twice my size, I hauled her out of the house, threw her in the car, drove a block away and called our social worker and the cops. The police convinced the man to give up the gun while the social worker convinced the wife to send her husband to the hospital for observation. Fortunately the man was quite debilitated so he couldn't put up much of a fight. We ultimately admitted this patient to a nursing home for his own safety, as he insisted that no matter what we did he would find a way to kill himself. In the end, he didn't kill himself and he did die peacefully.

OCCASIONALLY, I WILL care for a cancer patient who begs me to kill them. It breaks my heart when I hear that. I want to reach out and hold them close, comfort them and assure them with every fiber of my being that it will be okay. I understand the pain they are experiencing and the desperation they are feeling. I tell them I can't kill them, that even if it wasn't against the law, I wouldn't kill them. What I can do is give them medication that will help ease the pain and any other symptoms they may experience. I assure them that if things get bad enough, I can put them out altogether so they'll sleep through the worst of it. Most patients and their families are pretty accepting and all we can do is hope for the best.

At the opposite end of the spectrum, there's always the well-meaning neighbor who walks in the door under the guise of helping and blurts out in front of the family, "Oh, you're the hospice nurse? Hospice killed my dad." Hospice nurses don't kill people.

Families experience enough guilt without hearing those words, and I hear those exact words more often than you'd think. Hospice is not in the business of killing people. Our patients are dying of a terminal illness, any illness for which there is no cure, no respite, no remission, and the outcome of which is inevitably death. Our job is to make the inevitable as comfortable as possible. We don't kill people. Death kills people

He's Got His Own

I GOT A call one day to meet with the court-appointed legal guardian for an elderly man. We met in front of the home of her *ward*. She was hoping I could convince him to accept hospice services. The gentleman was dying of lung and laryngeal cancer and it had spread to his head and neck. He'd been sick a long time and the place had obviously been neglected. She and I entered his home together. The front door opened straight into the living room and the potential patient was sitting on a couch facing me. There wasn't much left of him.

Head and neck cancer and the results of a surgical intervention are disturbing. It's an ugly kind of surgery. To call it disfiguring is a gross understatement. Most of the right side of the man's jaw, cheek and neck were gone. His right eye drooped. He was unable to blink due to nerve damage and tears streamed down what was left of his ravaged right cheek. His nose was half-gone and his head fell to the right at an impossible angle, as the neck muscles and a portion of his clavicle on the right had all been removed. His body was skeletal. He had obviously once been a robust man, but now the skin hung from his bones like old raggedy clothes on a scarecrow. He took one look at me and even in his weakened state attempted to bolt, although his pace was about that of a tortoise and he didn't get far before his guardian caught him and ushered him back to the couch.

"No nurses," he insisted through the vibrating mechanism inserted into his tracheotomy.

All I could think was, "Oh boy."

The gentleman needed help desperately. He lived alone. Apparently he lived on the couch and there was no one to cook for him, to help him to the bathroom, to bathe him or clean him up. His pain was off the charts, but he didn't want pain medication. He didn't want hospice and he didn't want a nurse. He equated us with death and I guess he had that right. When you are dying and you refuse to go to the hospital, your physician often calls hospice. The man said he wanted to be left alone. I asked if that meant he was willing to die alone, you know, just fall on the floor and die all alone and someone would come find him whenever. He said, "Yes."

I took his hand and though he pulled away at first, he finally looked directly up at me and I asked him again if he wanted to be left alone. His answer didn't change.

His guardian walked me out. We stood on the front porch and talked for a long time. I offered to let her off the hook. I said I could call Adult Protective Services for her. Not only did she decline, in all honesty it didn't seem the right thing to do. If he wanted to die by himself, who was I to question that? Someone would find him.

His guardian promised to look in on him daily as did his neighbor. Very likely one of them would find him dead and call 9-1-1. That's about all they could do. I did suggest that at the very least, they figure out a way to convince him to allow a hired caregiver in to help with meals and toileting, and I advised them to go to the nearest medical supply store to buy or rent a bedside commode and maybe see if they could get him to take an occasional dose of morphine.

A week passed and another call came in regarding this gentleman. I again paid a visit to the home. The guardian had made bit of progress in that the gentleman had agreed to a hired caregiver, a lovely young Filipino girl with a very gentle demeanor. As I walked in the door, I saw that he held her hand in a death grip, as if she was his lifeline and his ship was sinking fast. The guardian was hoping he'd changed his mind and would now accept hospice services. She'd failed to notice that he'd chained himself to the couch. He'd actually found a long chain, like the kind you use to tow something behind your car. He'd wrapped it around his waist several times and then somehow managed to run it through a hole he'd cut in the back of the couch, and he'd locked it all together with a heavy padlock. I burst out laughing. He may not have been able to hold his head up, and he slumped against his caregiver like a spineless bag of bones, but he was so proud of what he'd done with that chain.

"No nurses," he said again. "I've got all I need right here."

I couldn't stop smiling. All I could say was, "You go, Mr. Black!" To this day I smile when I picture that chain wrapped around his waist.

At the request of his doctor, I did check on him one last time and I found him to be happy and very much at peace. He died quietly on his couch a day or so later, on his own terms.

The Ants Go Marching

MR. ANDREWS WAS kind of a hand-me-down from a nurse whose area changed. I adored him. She mentioned in passing that he had an *ant problem* and I assumed she meant there were ants in the house. No big deal, I'd had problems with them myself, especially during the rainy season. Anyway, he was dying of skin cancer that had metastasized to almost every organ in his body. It's a sad thing, but also far too common. I've admitted many elderly people who ignored an unusual mole or sore until they were dying of it.

Mr. Andrews had squamous cell carcinoma all over his body. He had a particularly ugly, large, necrotic wound on the top of his head. According to the doctor's report, it was in the layers of the skin only. Supposedly it had not invaded the skull and the brain. From the appearance of the wound, one might think differently.

Mr. Andrews liked to sleep in so I always arrived at his home around eleven a.m. His stepson had taken leave from his job to care for him on weekdays, along with a hired caregiver, and Mr. Andrew's two daughters alternated weekends. The four of them were wonderful loving caregivers and I never worried about neglect or my patient's safety.

On the morning in question, Mr. Andrew's stepson

greeted me at the door as usual. The patient was still asleep. I decided to take a peek and see if I could rouse him because I had a very full day ahead of me. The room was dim. The only light came from a single window covered with a thick dark green drape. Nonetheless, I noticed something odd about my patient's head. His skin appeared to be moving. I squinted and inched closer. No, it wasn't possible. I didn't believe my eyes. I had to be mistaken. I flipped on the light.

Oh my God! I was right! A river of ants was moving in and out of my patient's scalp wound. There were thousands, millions of them, climbing down the wall, up the bed, over the pillow, up the side of his head, burrowing under the dressing and then back the same way they came in, carrying pieces of my patient's necrotic scalp in their jaws.

Horrified, I flapped my arms like some deranged waterfowl, hopping up and down, screaming at the top of my lungs. The stepson and caregiver came running. Mr. Andrews, who was as deaf as a post, opened his eyes and smiled up at us. I could only point, speechless.

Using a syringe and sterile saline, I flushed the ants out of the deep scalp wound while the other two vacuumed furiously. When I inspected the wound, I was floored. It was amazing. In one night, the ants had managed to remove all the necrotic tissue and Mr. Andrews hadn't felt a thing. The wound bed was a very healthy pink. How disgustingly interesting!

I wondered why the ants were attracted to the wound in the first place. I suppose they could have been attracted by the smell of decaying flesh, except the wound didn't have much of an odor, at least to a human. The cancer had eaten its way clear down to the skull, and I started to think that maybe it had eroded into the skull and Mr. Andrews might have been leaking cerebrospinal fluid. Cerebrospinal fluid is sweet. It contains a lot of glucose, sugar. Ants love sugar. There you go. Regardless, I was horrified yet grateful to the ants. They saved Mr. Andrews an uncomfortable month of gradual wound debridement at my hands.

Anyway, we needed to deal with the *ant problem*. Since the family didn't believe in pesticides and neither do I, we went on a quest to find the nest and patch up their access route into the house. It was kind of fun and we were pretty successful with our judicious use of cayenne pepper, non-stick cooking spray and putty. Mr. Andrews was never again a meal, though I did find an occasional ant on a hopeful exploratory foray into the bedroom. After all, he was a very sweet man.

Sweet Surrender

THE ARTIST SPENT his last few hours on earth with his wife and me. His home was a museum, all his pieces displayed to their best advantage. He worked in a variety of mediums, oils, pastels, watercolors, clay, bronze, glass. The glasswork was especially beautiful. The rooms in his home were filled with vividly colored lamps and hanging chandeliers, splitting sunlight and reflecting rainbows into every corner.

The day before the Artist died, his entire family came to celebrate his seventieth birthday. It was a good day. He was awake and able to speak a few words to everyone he cared about. He said goodbye to his loved ones and predicted that he would die the next day at two p.m. He told them not to come back for the death. I came instead.

I arrived at eleven in the morning in case his timing was a little off. The Artist was indeed dying. He was unconscious and his breathing was noisy, heavy and irregular. His wife sat near the hospital bed in a rocking chair, quietly knitting away. I wandered through the house and yard, appreciating my patient's incredible talent while at the same time keeping an ear tuned to pauses in his respirations.

The garden was really something. The Artist had nestled small bronze sculptures in unexpected places and in my wanderings I stumbled upon them by accident as he intended. He'd designed the garden around an idea of organized chaos. I loved it. He'd captured the essence of life, at least as I see it, chaotic and always unexpected, with a sort of underlying organizational framework.

I eventually stopped my meanderings and sat in a chair for the remainder of the death watch. His wife and I waited in silence, each of us wrapped in our own thoughts as we almost absently watched the uneven rise and fall of his chest. When his respirations would pause, we each held our breath. When he noisily sucked in air, we exhaled. Out of the corner of my eye, I kept track of the wall clock ticking off the minutes, wondering if his prediction would prove accurate.

The house was peaceful, the shades drawn to keep things quiet, though the windows were open as the summer day was perfect, cool and clear. It was one of the softest afternoons I've ever spent, possibly the sweetest surrender to death I've ever witnessed. About one-thirty the artist's breathing slowed, the pauses grew longer. We kept watch even though I believe strongly in the saying, *a watched pot never boils*. At two o'clock on the nose, the Artist stopped breathing and died.

The wife and I sat there a few more minutes in silence. At last she said, "That's it then."

I nodded in agreement. "He did well."

"He did very well," she said.

Mary

MARY HAD BEEN dying for a week, in a coma, unresponsive to verbal and tactile stimuli. I didn't know Mary and had never before made a visit, but from the report I received, I assumed this would be her last day and I would be her last nurse. As it turned out, I was the last nurse to see her but the visit was far from what I expected.

As I stepped onto the old fashioned wooden veranda and approached the front door, I was surprised to hear singing coming from inside the house. I knocked and an East Indian woman, Mary's hired caregiver, opened the door. She was grinning from ear to ear. Her grin made her look just like the Cheshire cat from *Alice In Wonderland*. I stepped into the front room, the room that contained the hospital bed, the oxygen equipment and the patient.

There sat my patient, propped up on pillows and looking for all the world like the Queen of England, conversing animatedly with two church ladies who had come to pray over what they assumed would be her dying body. My mouth dropped open. I had just managed to stammer out a greeting to Mary when I noticed Mary's caregiver motioning me into the kitchen. I excused myself in Mary's general direction, she had been blind for ten years, and she replied with a genial wave, then returned her attention to her guests.

The caregiver could barely suppress her excitement over the morning's events. Apparently, she'd cleaned and changed Mary first thing, as usual, and Mary had been as unresponsive as she'd been every morning for the past week. Then she went into the kitchen to heat up a frozen cinnamon roll for her own breakfast. The woman was astonished to hear a voice cry out from the living room, "That smells real good! I'd like one of those!"

The caregiver nearly fainted. She thought she was hearing a ghost. Terrified, she peeked around the corner and found Mary wide awake, smacking her lips. The caregiver tore the cinnamon roll into pieces and fed Mary one piece at a time. She said Mary wolfed it down and claimed it was the best thing she'd ever tasted. Then Mary asked for some tea, so the caregiver brewed a pot of tea, added a little sugar and cooled it down for her. Mary drank the entire pot.

Amazed, I returned to the front room. Mary's guests were just saying their goodbyes and I showed them out. I turned to Mary and asked her a few questions, how was she feeling and so on. She reported that she had never felt better and she proceeded to sing me a song the likes of which I've never heard before or since.

Mary's voice was strong and incredibly beautiful and she sounded much younger than her eighty-some years. Odd as it seems, although I listened carefully in silence, the words of her song escaped me even as I heard them. The lyrics seemed slippery somehow and I couldn't grasp exactly what she was singing. Nor could I manage any response. Mary's song seemed to filter through me and then it sort of faded away above my head like breath on a cold winter night. It was a very other-worldly experience. I saw that it affected her caregiver the same way. She stood in the doorway between the living room and the kitchen. I think her feet were rooted to the spot.

We were silent for a few moments. Finally, I shook my head, shaking off an enchantment, and I gathered my thoughts. I gazed around the room. Even though Mary was blind she had quite a display of baseball memorabilia, more specifically, San Francisco Giants collectibles. She also had one Oakland A's bobble head on her mantle. My husband is a big baseball fan and has season tickets to the Giants, so of course, after complimenting her on her song, to break the ice I asked about her collection and I mentioned the A's bobble head. Her response was priceless.

Mary exclaimed, "Who the hell put that up there!?! I'm a Giants fan! Get rid of that A's bobble-head!"

So of course I then had to follow up with, "Well, you'll be happy to know that Bonds just hit his six hundredth homerun last night. My husband and my daughter were at the game."

To which Mary replied, without missing a beat, "Why didn't someone wake me up out of my coma to tell me?"

I laughed so hard I nearly wet my pants.

At that moment I noticed our hospice Home Health Aide coming up the walk. The caregiver and I raced each other to the door. I won.

"Dee," I cried throwing the door wide open, "you are not going to believe this!"

Dee took one look at Mary and her response was the same as mine. I stuck a finger under her chin and closed her mouth for her. Mary called out her name and Dee shook her head in disbelief. She said, "Now I've seen everything."

All business, Dee asked Mary if she wanted a bath and she nodded and asked for a shampoo and a manicure to boot. I decided it was time to call the next of kin and notify her of this interesting turn of events.

Mary had no children but she had a niece whom she had raised as her own daughter and they were very close. I was able to reach the niece at her real estate office and I asked her to come by as soon as possible. I told her that Mary was awake. I heard a crash through the receiver as her phone hit the floor. She never did hang it up.

I assisted Dee with Mary's personal care, while Mary sang and chatted. Abruptly, she turned to Dee and in a very matter of fact way said, "I need a man."

Dee stopped dead. "You need a man?"

"Yes, I need a man," was Mary's deadpan reply.

Dee, turning to an old wedding photo behind her on a chest asked, "What about your husband?"

"Oh, him! I just saw him when I was dead and I don't want him anymore!"

An eyebrow raised, Dee asked, "You don't want him

anymore?"

"Hell no. I never wanted him when I was alive! I want a different man."

"You want a different man? You want me to just walk outside and pick you up a man? Any man?"

"That'd be fine with me!"

Through our giggles, Dee and I managed to make Mary presentable. We got her propped back up on her pillows and she lay there, beaming. I would describe her as beaming beatifically but she was not one-hundred percent saint. She was more like a wonderfully wrinkled old Puck or Bacchus. She stated emphatically that this was the happiest moment of her life and promptly asked if there was any beer in the fridge. This elicited another chorus of giggles from Dee, the caregiver and me, but we all trooped dutifully into the kitchen to raid the fridge and yes, there was indeed a single bottle of ice cold beer. I asked her if she wanted it in the bottle or if she'd prefer a glass. I'm sure you already know the answer to that question. I helped her hold the bottle and bring it to her lips.

Mary *loved* the beer, the weight of the glass bottle in her hand, the cold condensation against her skin, the bittersweet malt taste on her tongue and the icy burn of the liquid down her throat. I think I can say that I will never again, as long as I live, see anyone drink a beer with such pleasure. We watched in reverent silence.

There are no words to describe what we all saw. It was as if we were witness to a pure act, the pure act of drinking a pure beer. The moment was distilled to the very essence of drinking a cold beer and in that very Zen moment, all four of us in the room found ourselves standing with one foot in heaven.

Mary smacked her lips and said, "That's good beer!"

Oh, yes, it was indeed.

Mary's niece arrived just as Mary finished her beer.

Tears flowed then laughter erupted as Mary ordered her to get pen and paper. She barked, "Write this down!"

Her niece sat dutifully at the head of the bed, recording Mary's very specific instructions regarding her funeral, what she wanted to be buried in, what hymns she wanted sung, what psalms she wanted read and what food she wanted served at the reception. She did expect a reception.

The niece gave me a hug and whispered, "What a gift!"

Mary slipped back into a coma several hours later and died comfortably early the next morning.

An Unusual Postscript

THREE YEARS LATER I encountered Mary's niece at the bedside of another patient, her cousin who was dying of liver failure. Small world! I thought I recognized her, but it wasn't until she began speaking of her aunt's death that I was able to put her into the right context.

She began to talk to me about Mary's last day and the hospice nurse who visited and I exclaimed, "That was me!"

Her niece described everything that happened after I left. She said Mary wanted a piper to play *Amazing Grace* at her service and it had to be an Irish piper, not a Scottish piper, God forbid!

Mary carried on conversations all day with people, seen and unseen, sometimes interrupting her conversation with her niece to speak with her previously deceased sisters, who she claimed were still arguing after death.

At some point in the middle of the night during the bedside vigil, Mary's niece lit a candle for her and told her, "When the candle goes out, your soul can move on."

She said it was only a small votive that should have burned for an hour or so but it continued to burn long after the wax had disappeared and she could no longer see any wick.

Finally, very fatigued, she got up and went into the kitchen to make herself a cup of tea. When she returned to the front room a few minutes later, the candle had gone out and Mary had died. She told me she thinks about Mary's beautiful death frequently. I told her I do, too.

Mary's brief return to the land of the living was truly a rare gift, but Mary is not the only patient of mine to return from the dead. A number of other patients have described their visions of heaven as they neared the end of life. However, Mary was able to communicate her experience more vividly than most. The interesting thing is she was blind, yet she could see and speak with the dead people surrounding her that last day. It doesn't surprise me. All kinds of weird things happen when a patient is near death.

5: Near Death

My Own Story

HERE IS THE story of my own near death experience. When I come right down to it, it's hard to talk about. The only person who knew the whole story was my best friend, Cheryl, and she died several years ago of heart failure. It's only been relatively recently that I've felt comfortable enough to discuss what happened. Because, you know, you lay it all out there, open yourself up and make yourself vulnerable, and people think you're nuts, or faking, or opposed to religion, or trying to cash in, or something.

Let me give you some background. I grew up the eldest child in a secular, politically active, Jewish family. All through my childhood and most of my early adulthood, my father identified himself as a devout atheist. He frequently boasted that he didn't believe in God, yet he could still be a Jew. My mother can best be described as an agnostic. Despite the fact that she sets a mean Passover table, I don't believe she has enough understanding of Judaism, or any other religion, to participate in a serious discussion of comparative religions if her life depended upon it. I can't remember ever even hearing her discuss her concept of God or heaven or life after death.

In fact, it seemed as if God was only mentioned in our household when His existence was being negated. Even as a small child, I repeatedly heard the following litany, or mantra, "There is no God. There is no heaven. There is no hell. Life on earth is an accident. Our lives are as insignificant as a microscopic speck of dust in the universe. After you die, you're buried and the worms eat you. There is *nothing* after death."

I lay awake at night from the age of three on, terrified of the *nothing* that lay in store for me when I died.

I was given an extensive orthodox Jewish education by a series of rabbis. They ranged from a gentle man who barely spoke English, to a pedophile, to a brilliant scholar who prided himself on his secular humanism and his atheism. Such was my unwitting background on the day in question.

My accident happened in early spring. I was sixteen years old and I was riding Heather, my quarter horse. My sisters had accompanied me to Charlie's ranch where we boarded the horse.

Charlie owned hundreds of hilly acres of undeveloped forest and unfenced pastureland halfway between Council Bluffs and Missouri Valley, Iowa. His place was a rider's dream. Knowing my obsession with horses, when my dad did some legal work for Charlie, he waved his usual legal fees in exchange for a horse. When I acquired Heather, she was a green-broke two year old. At the time of the accident she was four, and she'd turned into a very dependable mount.

Shortly after I became a horse owner my best friend, Cheryl, talked her dad into buying a horse, so we spent every spare minute together on horseback. I had confidence in Heather. I believed I could ride her anywhere.

On this particular day Cheryl was sick with a bad cold, so I rode alone. My youngest sister hung out with Charlie

and the ranch hands. My middle sister stayed in the car
with the windows rolled up. She's allergic to horses. As
usual, I rode bareback, which when you come right down
to it, is probably what saved my life. Given what occurred
later, had I used a saddle the saddle horn very likely would
have ruptured my liver or spleen or my aorta.

I'd ridden the trails for over an hour when it occurred
to me that my sisters must be getting pretty bored, so I
turned and headed back to the barn. There had been a
commotion near the barn before I took off. A woman who
owned a white Arabian mare had argued with her husband
about the horse. He'd insisted upon riding the horse and
his wife insisted he couldn't. The Arabian was my least favorite horse stabled at the ranch. Her temperament left a
lot to be desired. She spooked easily, not to mention the
annoying and dangerous habit she'd acquired of biting or
kicking anything within striking distance. But by the time I
made my way back, I'd forgotten all about the incident.

As I rode down the hill behind the barn, I stopped. I
moved my horse off the main trail, up onto a small rise. I
sat quietly on her back and simply enjoyed the view of the
valley. I think there is nothing like being on the back of a
horse. Nothing like it in the entire world, I mean, as long as
it's a good horse and as long as you love horses as much as
I do.

Out of nowhere, the woman's husband on the Arabian
mare he wasn't supposed to be riding, raced around a corner behind me and turned down the main trail toward the
barn. We had a commonsense rule at the ranch, no racing
toward the barn. It's an obvious safety rule that also keeps
the horses from becoming barn sour. The guy was yelling
his head off and holding onto the saddle horn for dear life,
the horse completely out of control. I remained calm.
There was plenty of room on the main trail and I was way
off to the side. All I had to do was sit quiet and let him

pass.

As he got closer, his horse veered my way and Heather started to dance. At that point, I had nowhere to go. There was a drop off on three sides of the rise. I felt sure the Arabian would see the barn and keep to the main trail. I definitely did not want to move directly into her path. But she kept coming at me with the rider flapping wildly on her back.

Being sixteen and innately over-confident, I figured I could control the situation. Afterwards, I realized I should have gotten off my horse and just let her go. But at that moment, I was actually a little afraid to get off Heather. The Arabian might trample me to death. I was also concerned someone would be injured by two runaway horses. No one near the barn had yet realized what was happening.

As the Arabian galloped toward us, Heather reared. I could have jumped off then, but I didn't. I dropped the reins and grabbed her mane when she reared again, but this time she stepped backward off the rise and flipped, head over heels, landing on top of me.

Events occurred in slow motion. We fell. I hit the dirt and I saw her chestnut back hurtling toward me. In an instant, every single cell in my body knew without a doubt that I was dead, and in that instant I left my body. I floated maybe thirty feet up in the air and watched the scene unfold before me.

Heather fell between my legs and across my torso, breaking my pelvis and crushing my chest and several vertebrae in my back. My body was tossed like a rag doll. It laid there, eyes closed, lifeless. I could not have cared less. From where I watched my body didn't matter a thing to me, not a single thing. I felt complete indifference to the fact that I was dying.

As I continued to hover above everyone, I saw my little sister scream and cover her face with her hands. I saw the look of shock on my middle sister's face through the car window. I watched the Arabian race into the barn, scattering people and horses in every direction. Heather righted herself and then followed the Arabian down the main trail. I watched as Charlie ran from the barn, glanced up the hill, grabbed Heather's reins, threw himself onto her back and headed for me. I didn't care. I was long gone. I had only one regret, I wished my sisters didn't have to see me die.

All the time I watched someone was beside me. I seemed to know him, or at the very least, expect him. In other words, I wasn't surprised by his presence. A great many things were happening at once, but that was okay, I had all the time in the world, or possibly no time since time didn't seem to be a factor in my life any longer. Maybe I was outside of time. Maybe it didn't exist for me.

As I floated a three-dimensional vision of my life began to unfold before me. I could see and feel the events of my life from my own perspective, but at the same time I could also feel the impact I had on others. If I hurt someone, I hurt myself. If I was kind to someone, I felt their happiness as my own. The vision itself was neutral, as was my companion. I realized I wasn't being judged; I *was* the judge. I judged my own life. Any wrongs I'd done to others, I did to myself. Any pain I'd caused anyone, no matter how slight, I felt it. It was a life altering experience.

At the same time, it seemed as if the universe lay exposed before me. I had no more questions. All those nagging questions like, *why am I here, what is the meaning of life, what happens after death?* They had all vanished from my mind. Everything made sense. I no longer know *what* made sense, but I knew then. In other words, I don't remember the answers, I forgot them as soon as I was alive again, but I remember very clearly that I knew the answers to those questions when I was dead.

My companion with me took me on a journey. We held hands and surfed on a wave of light. It was totally cool because we went faster and faster until we reached what I guess would be the speed of light. Before we reached the speed of light things were still separate. I could differentiate one object from another. After we reached the speed of light, or whatever the barrier was, we crossed a threshold and on the other side everything became one thing, one undifferentiated thing that contained all of life.

My companion spoke with me while we surfed. He said a great many things but I only remember one. I remember that one thing because he took his finger and wrote it in my heart.

He said, "All paths lead to truth. All roads lead to God."

Just then we stood within a perfect unblemished white light that took up my entire field of vision. The light was neither hot nor cold. It was the brightest thing I've ever seen, yet I could look upon it without difficulty. The light was alive. It held me and I felt comforted, surrounded by *love*. The best way I can describe the sensation is to say that I was cradled in the arms of God even though He doesn't have arms. Words are inadequate, but words are all I have.

From his lap, I gazed rapturously at the vibrant colors of heaven, watching a parade of figures approach, when a voice suddenly said, "You didn't die, you have to go back."

I pleaded, "No! No! No! Don't send me back! I don't want to go back! Please don't send me back!"

Immediately I was sucked into some kind of vortex and found myself right above my body. The same person who had taken me surfing on the wave of light accompanied me.

I cried out one more time, "Please don't send me back, I'll feel pain!"

I swear I howled that last part. But he sent me back.

The moment I entered my body was terrifying. I was sucked in from underneath and hit the inside of my face. Imagine being trapped in a casket and pounding on the inside of the lid, that's exactly how I felt. The sense of claustrophobia was unimaginable. I struggled desperately within my own body. To all outside appearances, my body didn't move while inside, I thrashed about, panic-stricken. Suddenly my companion was with me. He held my arms and gently smoothed me into myself. We meshed and I became one with my body. I was alive again.

For a moment I couldn't remember how to do any-thing, or how to work anything, how to move, how to speak. I felt someone kneeling above me and I managed to crack open one eye. It was Charlie. I croaked out his name, my voice sounding odd and foreign to me.

He started to cry. "Thank God! Thank God!"

Then Charlie did something you are never supposed to do in this situation, he threw me over the back of my horse with him and galloped to the barn. He tossed Heather's reins to one of the stable hands, laid me in the back seat of the car and drove us all home. We passed the hospital on the way. He was pretty panicked, I guess. I ended up out of commission for about six months but I made a complete recovery.

Is this experience why I ultimately became a hospice nurse? I don't know for sure but I think it's what makes me a good hospice nurse. The only thing I know with certainty is that in the end, everything will work out fine. And by the way, I want a Scottish piper to play *Amazing Grace*, not an Irish one.

Questions and Answers

Am I religious?

I identify as Jewish but I have deep spiritual beliefs that extend beyond the boundaries of traditional Judaism, some of which could probably get me excommunicated. Am I religious in the usual sense of the word? No.

Do I believe in God?

Yes.

Do I believe in the existence of the soul?

Without question.

Do I believe in heaven?

Yes.

Do animals go to heaven?

They certainly go to mine.

Do I believe in hell?

Yes. To quote a line from the Charles Dickens classic *A Christmas Carol*, "I wear the chains I forged in life." I believe that what we do or fail to do in this life determines our experience in the next. What we do to others, we do to ourselves.

Rabbi Hillel said in the first century BCE, "That which is hateful to you, do not do to your fellow. That is the whole Torah. The rest is commentary. Go and learn."

The Buddha said, "Whatever, after due examination and analysis, you find to be kind, conducive to the good, the benefit, the welfare of all beings, believe and cling to that doctrine and take it as your guide."

Muhammad said, "Whoever is kind to His creatures, God is kind to him. Therefore, be kind to man on earth, whether good or bad, and being kind to the bad, is to withhold him from badness, thus in heaven you will be treated kindly."

From the sayings of Lao-Tzu and *The Way of the Tao*, "To the good I would be good. To the not good, I would also be good in order to make them good."

Voltaire said, "Every man is guilty of all the good he did not do."

As Jesus stated so succinctly, "Judge not, that you may not be judged. For with what judgment you judge, you shall be judged and with what measure you mete, it shall be measured to you again." And, "Do unto others as you would have them do unto you."

Do I aspire to perfection?

No. It's simply not possible because I'm human and therefore inherently and wonderfully flawed. I try to be good and frankly, sometimes that can be a stretch. Besides, if I was perfect, why would I bother with all this life-stuff in the first place? Again, to quote Voltaire, "The perfect is the enemy of the good." If I strive too hard for perfection, I might just bypass the good altogether.

Do I pray?

Yes. Every minute of every day. I view every action as a prayer.

Have I seen ghosts?

Yes. Next question.

How can I do this kind of work? Isn't it depressing?

While hospice work can be awfully sad, it's never depressing. After working with hospice, there's no other kind of nursing I want to do. Death is totally real, definitely unambiguous and for the most part, it brings out the best in people, occasionally the worst, but usually the best. When someone is dying, the superficial falls away. Every moment, no matter how challenging, is precious because it will never come again. Of primary importance to both the patient and the family are the relationships, the memories, good and bad, and hopefully, love. Nobody cares anymore if they look fat in jeans, except for one patient who told me, "There's an up-side to cancer. I've lost sixty pounds and I've received so many compliments!" She was an aberration. Almost all my patients focus on connecting with the people who mean the most and, if possible, tying off loose ends. If I have a patient who is unable to communicate, due to a brain injury or dementia, it's the family that attempts to make the final transition from life to the acceptance of death, then cut the ties and set their loved one free.

Doesn't accepting hospice mean that the patient is giving up hope?

No, not at all. It means you're accepting the fact that you or a loved one has a terminal illness. Often patients on hospice actually live longer and suffer less discomfort than patients who die while undergoing treatment. It's a matter of changing focus, a shift from clinging to life no matter what the cost, to enjoying the things you can enjoy while hoping and praying for a good death.

A hospice patient can always decide to seek additional treatment, but in that case they are usually discharged from hospice, as insurance companies and Medicare will not pay for both hospice care and treatment. A patient can remain on hospice if they elect to pay for additional treatment out of pocket, or sometimes if they receive palliative care. Palliative care usually involves either chemo-therapy or radiation that is provided to help control symptoms such as pain and nausea. Either or both can be helpful in shrinking a tumor mass. Palliative care is not curative.

Will the patient get addicted to the pain medication?

Who cares? The patient will be dead in a few weeks anyway. I'm not trying to make light of the subject, but I do get that question all the time. Yes, a lot of the medications we use with hospice patients are addictive, but so what? Most patients don't live long enough for addiction to become an issue and even if they do live for a while, isn't pain control the most important consideration? Cancer pain can be the worst kind of pain. If medications are used properly they control the pain and allow the person to function as well as they can for the time they have left. That is not drug addiction.

Drug addiction is when you use the drugs simply to get high. Hospice in the United States uses a lot of morphine, morphine derivatives, methadone and various synthetic pain relievers with pretty good success. A few countries have legalized heroin for use specifically with cancer patients and hospice patients. Some studies indicate it can be quite effective for pain control and it has fewer side effects than morphine. However, heroin is illegal in the United States and I believe the same results can be achieved with morphine.

Who pays for hospice care?

Your tax dollars! Actually, the best thing about Medicare is the generous Hospice Benefit. Medicare, Medicaid, or Medical in our case, all pay for hospice services. Most private insurance companies also have a Hospice Benefit paid out at about the same rate as Medicare. The daily rate covers everything hospice provides, including nursing visits, home health aide services, appointments with the Medical Social Worker and chaplain, all medications related to comfort, and all equipment and supplies necessary to keep the patient safe, clean and comfortable. Most hospices also have a charitable foundation that allows them to provide care for patients without insurance. No one is ever billed for hospice services.

Is the patient dying?

Yes. A surprising number of families ask me not to talk to the patient about death. I'm even asked to keep quiet about the fact that I'm a hospice nurse. "Just tell him you're here to give him some extra attention." I've got news for you, your father, your mother, your sister, your brother, they already know. In their heart, they know. I'm willing to keep it on the down-low for a while, but they almost always ask and then I'm honest. I think when you are dying and you ask *that* question the least you deserve is an honest answer. People have things they need to finish up, even if it's something as simple as drinking a beer. Not a single patient has ever been angry with me for telling them the truth.

When will the patient die?

I have no idea. No, that's not true. When it comes to hospice patients I can usually call it pretty close. Even though it's not an exact science, my predictions are sometimes frighteningly accurate. Before I read the book *Blink, The Power of Thinking Without Thinking*, by Malcolm Gladwell, I had no idea how I did it. After reading the book, I think it's mostly because I'm able to read subtle cues and signs that most people miss. Plus I've always been a good guesser. I can usually give families a rough estimate. Generally speaking, hospice nurses are pretty tuned into the dying process and most are pretty accurate with their guestimates.

Do people on hospice ever "not die?"

Absolutely. Sometimes patients live for years, on or

off hospice. Sometimes their condition improves so dramatically that they graduate from hospice. They may be readmitted at some future date, but in the meantime we forget all about them.

One of the reasons elderly people occasionally improve on hospice, especially the folks in nursing homes, is that we give them more personalized attention. We manage their medications closely, eliminate meds that either aren't working or are contributing to the patient's ill health, and we treat pain and depression. Both pain and depression very often go unrecognized in the elderly. In addition, I've found that elderly patients can become deathly ill due to undiagnosed urinary tract infections. Once we clear up the infection they very often return to their previous level of functioning.

What is the worst disease to die of?

Wow. Big question. Dying is rarely easy unless you're one of those lucky people who unexpectedly dies in his sleep. I would have to say Congestive Heart Failure or Pulmonary Edema or Pulmonary Hypertension and Emphysema. The diseases are pretty much all the same in that you suffocate. I can't think of a worse feeling than slow suffocation or drowning in your own bodily fluids. Panic City all the time. These are really tough diseases to manage as you approach the end of your life. Morphine helps a lot with the shortness of breath and anxiety. There is no cure for the above conditions, but nonsmokers are less likely to develop them in the first place.

What's the easiest disease to die of?

Hands down, Acute Lymphocytic Leukemia, mostly because everything happens so fast. If untreated, my patients usually progress from diagnosis to death within two to four weeks. They grow weaker and weaker and then simply fall asleep. Pain doesn't seem to be as much of a factor as with other types of cancer, though we medicate patients just in case they experience some discomfort or shortness of breath due to anemia.

Does everyone who's dying have visions of heaven?

Not everyone. Most people, unless they are comatose, see *something*. At times my patients can describe very clearly what they are experiencing, other times it comes out a bit muddled. At one time or another in the last few weeks or days, almost every single patient who is able to speak tells me they receive visits from loved ones who have died before them, both beloved friends and family members.

One patient of mine who had been a flyer in World War II, frequently saw and spoke with many of the men from his squadron in his final days. I find it interesting that as they approach death, men who served in the war commonly visit with deceased friends from their squadron or unit. Those friends seem to be among the first to make a visit to a dying serviceman, even before deceased relatives arrive. Two of my uncles flew in World War II, one as a tail gunner and the other as a bombardier. I know that throughout their lives both my uncles remained very close with surviving members of their squadrons. I would venture to say that death does not break the significant bonds forged in this life.

Will the patient become incontinent before they die?

Chances are, no matter how much we all wish otherwise, yes. The only people spared that indignity are the lucky few who die suddenly, before they become bed bound. It's okay. Despite some initial embarrassment, nobody will think any less of the patient. Incontinence is simply a fact of hospice life and we all deal with it in a professional manner. Hospice personnel are very sensitive to the fact that our patients experience this loss of control. However, when you are dying, incontinence will bother you less than you think. Everyone has bigger fish to fry.

Am I afraid of dying?

Only a little, because I've seen how hard it can be. I'd be lying if I said not at all. Mostly I'm terrified of getting old and becoming infirm. I'm afraid someone will leave me lying in a bed on my back and never turn me. I hate sleeping on my back. I can just imagine the bed sores. I suffered through a nasty one in the hospital after my accident.

Since I'd prefer to avoid that scenario, I've devised a contingency plan. If I make it to eighty-nine and I'm still in pretty good shape, I'm applying for a permit to climb Mt. Everest. If I die in the attempt, oh well. My husband made an excellent suggestion. He said Mt. Hood would be closer, cheaper, every bit as treacherous, and the kids could bring the grandchildren by. I'm rethinking my original plan.

All kidding aside, the truth is, when I find myself stressing about the mundane, whether my bed is made, or my dishwasher emptied at some precise moment, my living room pillows arranged properly, or the dog hair vacuumed daily, I ask myself the following question, "When I'm on my deathbed, will those things matter?" The answer is inevitably, "No."

The Meadow

AS MR. BLUM'S daughter, Eva, packed for a long-planned vacation to Europe, we discussed the fact that her father would be gone by the time she returned to the States. Mr. Blum had already paid for the trip. It was a college graduation gift for Eva's twin sons. Eva was obviously supposed to accompany them. The original plan also included her dad. During Mr. Blum's more lucid moments, he urged her to go. I told her the same. There was really nothing more she could do.

Eva was racked with guilt. Who could have imagined when they planned this joyous celebration together that six months later her father would suffer a massive stroke and lie dying in a hospital bed in her living room? I reminded her that she'd hired a twenty-four hour caregiver and her sister had agreed to come by every day. I also promised Eva I would spend part of every day with her dad.

I remained with Mr. Blum the day Eva and her sons left. The young men tearfully kissed their grandfather goodbye, but they couldn't disguise their excitement as they hauled the luggage to the airport shuttle. I gave them each a hug and wished them well.

When I returned to the house, Eva was on her knees at her father's bedside, holding both his hands, asking him what to do. She wanted to go on the trip, but she didn't want to leave him. Mr. Blum roused himself and sat up with my assistance. Weak though he was, he gave her a hug and a kiss and ordered her to get into the shuttle.

Then he waggled his finger at me and said to Eva, "We won't be calling you if anything happens. When you get home will be soon enough."

Eva sobbed so hard she had to lean on me as we walked to the shuttle.

I said, "It will be okay. I'll take good care of him. I promise he will be fine."

"But, but . . ."

"No Eva," I said. "Go. He wants you to go. Do this for him. Do this for your boys. Whatever happens to your dad, whether it happens today, tomorrow, or the next day, there's nothing you can do. You already did your job. You've been a good daughter."

By the time the shuttle pulled away, even I was crying. When I returned to Mr. Blum's bedside, his eyes were closed but he knew I sat next to him. I read a book, waiting for the hired caregiver to return from her errands. Suddenly, with his good hand, Mr. Blum pointed to the wall by the foot of the bed.

"Can you see it?" he asked, his eyes open wide.

I guessed what he meant but I asked anyway, "See what?"

"The meadow," he replied, "the colors. Can you see them? Can you see how splendid they are?"

I turned and gazed at the wall. It was a big undecorated plain white wall. But I could feel a glow, like sunshine on my face.

"Is it heaven?" he asked in a small voice, sounding very much like a little boy.

"Yes," I assured him. "It's heaven."

Suddenly he sat forward, both arms outstretched, even his paralyzed right arm. His face shone with joy.

"What do you see?" I asked him.

"My wife is coming," he answered. "She's coming across the meadow."

"Do you want to go with her?" I asked. "Are you ready to go away with her?"

"Yes," he replied. Then he looked at me sternly. "Don't call my daughter," he said.

I smiled and drew my fingers across my mouth in a motion of zipping my lips. I helped him lay back against the pillows.

My arm still around his shoulders, Mr. Blum closed his eyes and died. A sense of peace descended upon the entire house. Tears squeezed out between my closed eyelids as I sat silently for the longest time, just holding him. I think I may have dozed off briefly. The caregiver roused me when she arrived loaded down with bags of groceries and rang the doorbell.

Arrangements had already been made for Mr. Blum's body, but I stayed with him to be sure that he was properly taken care of. Then I disposed of medications and supplies and had the equipment picked up. I didn't talk to Eva until she called me from the San Francisco airport two weeks later. Unfortunately her sister managed to contact her in France despite my suggestion that she hold off, so Eva already knew. We met at her house for coffee and I filled her in. The conversation was easier than I expected.

Eva and I walked arm in arm to have a look at the wall. We stood there for a long time in silence. Even a blank wall can be a doorway to heaven.

A Note To My Readers—

I've been on leave from hospice for nearly three years now. My reasons for saying goodbye to a job I loved were twofold. First and foremost our hospice computerized. Too much time was spent on a computer, far too little time at a patient's bedside. I did not become a nurse to interact with a computer screen. Not only is nursing an intensely hands-on experience, especially hospice nursing, it has always been collegial in the sense that hospice nurses provide support and expertise to other hospice nurses. With the introduction of computers our work could be done from home. Basically we worked in isolation. Although this saved our organization money it caused an increase in job-related stress for the staff.

Secondly, when the economy tanked our already poor county grew even more challenged. I became concerned for my safety. I was threatened with physical harm on two consecutive weekends, once by a patient's mentally ill son, and twice in a drug house. I had to face the fact that there was a real possibility I could be shot for the contents of my nursing bag. Of course I didn't carry drugs, but the assumption on the street is that hospice nurses do carry drugs. My husband was even more worried than I was and he insisted I take a leave of absence. I agreed.

I miss the work every single day.

About the Author

Heidi Telpner has been a nurse for over twenty-five years. She is currently on leave from hospice, pursuing her first dream—writing a novel.

Made in the USA
Lexington, KY
02 March 2014